Linda L. Miles'

PRACTICE DYNAMICS

Linda L. Miles

PRACTICE DYNAMICS

PennWell Books

**DENTAL
ECONOMICS**

PennWell Publishing Company
Tulsa, Oklahoma

Some passages in this book have been taken from articles of mine previously published in dental publications. Thanks go to Belinda Wilson of *Dental Management,* Ellen Dietz of *Dental Assisting,* and Dr. Arthur Williams of the *Journal of Dental Practice Management* for their spendid cooperation in this regard.

Thanks also to Jill Janov for permission to excerpt job interview questions from her booklet "Hiring Evaluating and Firing: Critical Skills for Managers and Supervisors."

Copyright © 1986 by
PennWell Publishing Company
1421 South Sheridan Road/P.O. Box 1260
Tulsa, OK 74101

Library of Congress cataloging in publication data

Miles, Linda L.
  Linda Miles'
  Practice dynamics.

  Includes index.
  1. Dental offices—Management.   2. Dentistry—Practice.
3. Success. I. Title.
RK3.M55   1986   617.6'0068   86-5904
ISBN 0-87814-301-7

Printed in the United States of America

  2   3   4   5   90   89   88

Acknowledgments

Thanks to . . .

My mom, the most caring and kind person I know, who loves people and taught me to do the same.

My dad, who taught me that hard work, dedication, and desire are essential for success.

My brother Ted and sisters Pat and Bobbie, who never made me have the "middle child syndrome."

My husband Don, the most supportive person on earth. Without his assistance, patience, and love I couldn't have followed my dream.

Our daughter LaDona, the joy of our life from Day One.

Our son David, our creative artist who will be "discovered" any day.

All my friends in the dental profession who believed in my theories long before anyone else did.

My staff—so loyal, dedicated, and appreciative. They make working for a living fun. To Lee, who completely "ran the ship" while I wrote the book, and to C. J., who worked side by side with me until our final manuscript went to press. To Carol and Pat, for assisting Lee during the time of writing.

Thanks also to . . .

My clients and their staff who built Dental Dynamics, Inc., through their many referrals.

Dr. Joe Dunlap, dental editor for PennWell Books, with whom I'm privileged to work. With his kind assistance, I *will* become a writer yet.

Frances Paget, friend and editor, who has helped me so much in the past.

My former dental employers who had the patience to allow me to grow in a positive direction. Each of them taught me so much, both clinically and personally.

And a special thanks . . .

My last dental employer, Dr. Richard S. Wilson of Richmond, Virginia. He taught me the art of appreciation for patients and dentistry. His enthusiasm inspired me to start Dental Dynamics, Inc. He was fully supportive in my desire to grow professionally. To him I will forever be grateful.

Linda L. Miles

Contents

Introduction

Welcome to the dynamic world of dentistry! I feel that dentistry should be fun, exciting, and rewarding for patients, dentists, and staff. I can't think of anything worse than going to work every day to a job you don't like. If you agree, you will enjoy this book.

While managing the office of Dr. R.S. Wilson in Richmond, Virginia, I served as president of the Richmond Metropolitan Dental Assistants Association. On my day off, I consulted with dentist friends of Dr. Wilson on business systems within their practices. I keenly remember the lack of enthusiasm in many of their offices compared to Dr. Wilson's. I soon realized that the happier offices were also the ones that were the most productive. That was when I began the pursuit of happiness in dentistry.

One day a young dentist with whom I was consulting said, "Your ideas are great and my staff members are very enthused. Have you ever thought of doing an all-day seminar for doctors and staff?" That was the beginning of my firm, Dental Dynamics, Inc. We are now a full-fledged speaking and dental consulting business—the largest in the Southeast

Consulting assignments in more than 300 offices have kept me aware of the accelerating changes that have occurred in the dental field in the past decade. For the most part, all offices share similar problems and frustrations. Out of all my experiences, I have defined four ingredients for success (the basis for Dental Dynamics, Inc.):

1. communication
2. organization
3. motivation
4. appreciation

Communication

Lack of communication within the office is an enormous handicap to growth. Noncommunication with patients is equally destructive. Even though I don't like the term "selling," communication is just that. The person answering the telephone "sells" the practice in the first 30 seconds of conversation. We "sell" to the patients by communicating their dental needs. Communication with the new patient is vitally important. We must ask questions and listen to the patient. People only buy what they want. As good communicators, we must make our patients want what they need. I have witnessed many instances in which cases were lost as a result of lack of communication or inability to close the sale.

Organization

Organization of the business area and systems is a problem in many practices. I feel the entire practice revolves around the business office—the hub of the practice. When it clicks, the entire office clicks. In most dental business facilities, the physical layout of the business office is wrong. It tends to be too small or in a corner of the office; or the appointment book, computer terminal, pegboard, or other piece of equipment is in the wrong place for maximum efficiency. It is amazing how smoothly the office begins to function when the physical layout is improved and the system is organized.

Motivation

Motivation is a gift we give ourselves. When we wake up in the morning, *we* decide if we are going to have a great or terrible day. As my friend Dr. Duane Schmidt, author of *3 Steps to the Million-Dollar Practice* and *Earn More–Work Less*, says, "When you program yourself to have a great day, no turkey can mess it up." Moods also affect motivation. We owe it to our co-workers to leave personal problems on the office doorstep so we can be at peak performance every day. A mood board in your staff lounge or lab is a fun way of staying aware of moods. Each team member, including the doctor, must sign in each morning by placing an applique beside his or her name on the mood board.

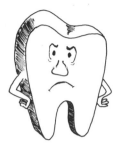

Today is not a good day,
I need some hugs

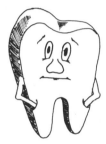

Today's an Okay day (too early—
I don't wake up until noon)

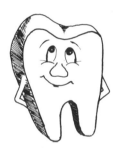

Today is a wonderful day

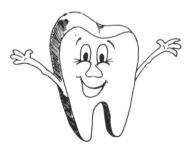

If I felt any better, I would
be arrested

Well-defined team incentives keep the motivation and morale in the office high and allow everyone to pull in the same direction at the same time.

Appreciation

I think it would be fair to say that 95 percent of the doctors and their staff in this country do not feel appreciated by their co-workers and patients. In order to receive appreciation, we must give it. Nothing makes a person feel better than a sincere compliment. I have seen offices double in production after they began practicing the art of appreciation.

Begin by telling patients how much you appreciate them and their referrals. Watch how many more referrals the practice receives.

Staff members should compliment the doctor and his or her dentistry in front of the patients. Such staff approval is a major factor in building patients' confidence in the dentist.

Similarly, doctors should compliment the staff in front of their patients and co-workers. Praise and apprecation are the greatest practice-builders in the world, and they don't cost a dime.

The success of Dental Dynamics, Inc. results from changes that have occurred in the practices that apply my four ingredients of success. Doctors report that it is wonderful to go to work in a "dynamicized" office where the staff members all get along and have a personal interest in the patients and the practice. Simply stated, happy people are productive people.

Staff members are amazed to find that managing the dental practice really can be fun and rewarding if everyone pitches in. They also report a positive change in their employers' attitudes which, ultimately, affect their own. Job attitudes affect personal attitudes. The quality of our off-duty hours improves quickly when we feel good about our work and co-workers. In addition, a positive job attitude causes others to view our job similarly—a point of special significance with a spouse.

After consulting and speaking for hundreds of dental groups, I felt I should write this book and share my observations, which have proven helpful to many dental practices. I don't have all the answers, nor will the ideas in this book fit every dental office. As I recommend in my presentations, you should attend several practice management courses, listen to different speakers, try to match the philosophy of the speaker with that which is desired, and then design a plan of action. What works best in one office may not work well in another.

This book can be used as a training manual for new employees or as a refresher course for those who are experiencing the beginning symptoms of burnout.

One of my goals is for every dental staff member who reads this book to realize the great importance of loyalty. It is a frequently overlooked trait in employees. When I changed my attitude from "me" to "we," my entire life changed. When I started thinking "What can I do for the practice?" rather than "What can the practice do for me?" I began to realize that you get out of a job or career exactly what you put into it.

If this book presents useful ideas, modifies your thinking, and warms your heart, it will fulfill my goal of sharing.

Chapter 1

Assembling
the Staff

One of the most important tasks confronting the new or experienced doctor is hiring a caring staff that will work well as a team.

In assembling the staff, whether it be the first employee or an addition to an existing staff, many factors come together to determine success or failure. As most dental practitioners who have hired in a hurry admit, "Haste makes waste." This chapter offers guidelines for assembling a staff that will reduce stress and help ensure success. Remember, interviewing and training are expensive processes, so there's wisdom in selecting staff members carefully. As H. Ross Perot, Chairman of the Board of Electronics Data Systems says, "Eagles don't flock; you must find them one at a time."

Advertising for Staff

The key to hiring good employees is to have a good selection of winners to choose from. The type of ad placed in the newspaper definitely affects the caliber of the applicants.

Some dentists' hiring methods remind me of the story about the farmer who lost his wife. After the shock of her passing subsided, he missed her so much he decided to place an ad for a new wife. It read as follows:

Wanted: Good farm wife (with tractor).
Please send picture (of tractor).

It is obvious the farmer was more interested in a farmhand than in a wife. Many dental ads are similarly misleading in that they make the job sound like a marshmallow position by using phrases such as "wonderful position," "excellent salary and benefits," "fantastic hours." These job descriptions attract losers who are looking for candy-coated jobs, not career-minded winners looking for challenges.

If the office wishes to hire only dynamic staff members, employment advertisements should contain phrases that attract winners such as: "Are you *caring* and *enthusiastic?* Do you enjoy a challenge in the health care profession? Are you *dependable* and *goal-oriented?*" These words attract job applicants who develop into great team members.

An advertisement listing the office telephone number has pros and cons. The pros include being able to screen the calls to determine the applicant's ability to converse over the phone. The cons are that (1) incoming applicant calls may interrupt normal tasks and (2) many unqualified applicants may call about the job.

A blind ad asks applicants to mail their résumé and a cover letter to a newspaper or post office box. Career-minded applicants have résumés and know how to compose good cover letters. Such data, of course, can be inflated to make applicants appear better than they are. But dental staff members must have initiative. Putting together a résumé and sending an individually composed letter are indications of this trait. It also gives the office an opportunity to scan the résumé and letter for misspelled words or poor sentence structure, indications of haste or insufficient education.

The following are examples of effective ads for dental office personnel. In each case, the ads have been structured (1) to attract the most desirable persons and (2) to help the prospective applicants screen themselves.

(1)   WANTED: Dental Assistant (part time). Are you an enthusiastic, experienced dental assistant with a caring manner? Are you dependable and organized? If so, please send résumé to Box 523, c/o this paper.

(2)   WANTED: Dental Business Assistant (full time). Do you have excellent communication skills over the telephone and in person? Are you enthusiastic, caring, and dependable? If you have experience with appointment book control, insurance, and bookkeeping and you like working in an office that appreciates staff, please send résumé and cover letter in own handwriting to Box 41, c/o this paper.

(3) WANTED: Dental Hygienist (full time). If you are enthusiastic, caring, and dependable and you enjoy a challenge in a patient-centered practice, please call 481-2276 between 10 and 12 A.M. only.

(4) WANTED: Dental Assistant. Seeking an exceptional team person. We focus on warmth, caring, and expert communication. Emphasis on personal development through continuing education, participation with other team members, and high achievement. Applicant should be career-minded, personally stable, and health-centered in lifestyle. Call 497-8611.[†]

Advertisement 1 is an example of a brief ad that deliberately omits office hours and location. If you list evening and Saturday hours, for instance, you may reduce the number of applicants by as much as three-fourths. The key to hiring successfully is to have many résumés from which to choose. Details can be worked out later. In fact, some of the greatest success stories in hiring have been with staff members who traveled 25 to 30 miles to a particular job. Hours and distances are minor factors if the match is right.

[†]Reprinted with permission of Jack I. Cherin, DMD, Virginia Beach, Virginia.

Advertisement 2 may seem lengthy, but I feel business assistants must have the most detailed ad. They not only should be good in business skills but in human skills as well. Too many offices concentrate on business skills only to learn subsequently that the new receptionist is not a "people person." Others put a "charming hostess" up front, and within weeks she is overwhelmed by the responsibilities of trying to please the doctor, staff, and patients. Shortly after that, she leaves. Spending a few extra dollars on an ad and then screening carefully will save you money and stress.

Advertisement 3 is an example of a short, positive ad that may also serve as a marketing device. When people move to new communities, they often read want ads. Reading that a dental office is "patient-centered" may lead to new patients—therefore, the telephone number should be listed. To keep phone interruptions to a minimum, list the doctor's private number and have someone come in from 10 A.M. to noon to take the calls and screen the applicants. This keeps the calls from interrupting activities at the front desk.

Advertisement 4 is positive and directed at a special, high-achievement person. The money invested in the length of the ad saves many dollars' worth of time sifting through unqualified applicants.

Other Sources of Prospects

Besides newspaper advertisements, other sources of auxiliary personnel include the following.

Local Dental Assistants and Hygiene Associations

Within these groups there is sometimes an employment chairperson or networking contact. Such individuals keep telephone numbers of staff seeking employment and a log of offices needing staff. This "matchmaker" is simply a contact person who provides services for which no fee is normally charged.

Dental Sales Representatives

This "through-the-grapevine" contact has proven very beneficial because sales representatives often know who is available, or will be available, before it is public knowledge.

For instance, a staff person may confide in a sales representative that she is contemplating a move. Subsequently, an office person three blocks away may say to the sales rep, "We're losing our number one assistant; be on the lookout for us." Bingo! Utilizing such contacts can save time and money by eliminating the ad process.

Technical Schools

This is an excellent source of prospective employees. Notify the schools that the office is interested in securing a past or upcoming graduate. The alumnae of these schools often place their names on the "available" lists when they are between positions, even after graduating.

Employment Agencies

Those that specialize in dental placement services can be very helpful, even though there is a fee involved. If their pool of temporary and permanent placements is strong, the chances are good for finding a qualified staff member.

Beware of agencies that have a pool of untrained, low-qualified, unskilled workers. These types of agencies often charge hefty fees and make no guarantees in their contracts. Read the contract closely, ask questions, and check the agency's track record by asking for the telephone numbers of three offices that have used their services. If the agency says their policy is not to divulge client's names, keep looking. All reputable firms have happy clients who say, "You may use our name as a satisfied client."

Other Dental Offices

This should be the last place to look for employees. Actively stealing another office's staff with promises of higher pay or better benefits is unethical. I have heard staff members ask, "If they would steal another office's staff, what else might they do that is unfair?"

However, if a staff member in office A is a friend of a hygienist in office B, the office A person is free to say, "Our hygienist is leaving in a month." And if the office B hygienist then expresses interest in working in office A, it is completely ethical for her to be interviewed. As long as active recruiting of another's staff has not occurred, no harm has been done. Getting a reputation for stealing staff is not a practice-builder in any sense.

Inexperienced Applicants

An applicant's lack of experience is not always a detriment. Some doctors say they would rather create new habits than break old ones. I feel attitude should be considered first. If the applicant has a great attitude, she or he can learn to do any job in the office.

Waitresses, for example, are a potential source of dental office personnel. Notice them when you are dining in nice restaurants. A waitress who cares about customers, smiles freely, and moves quickly and with dexterity may be receptive to the prospects of a career rather than a job. You may believe waitresses have such good incomes from tips that they could never be lured into an office position. But the fact is many would gladly exchange their weekend and evening hours for careers in health care fields. I always say, "Ask! Nothing ventured, nothing gained." Many dentists report that some of their best employees have come from this tip.

Interviewing Prospects

Set an interview appointment for all qualified persons who respond to the solicitations. It is wise to allow the present staff to have input in the hiring process. If a business staff person is being hired, have another business staff member take the top three applicants to lunch individually. If that is not possible, have a present staff member participate in the preliminary interview. I have found that hard-working, industrious staff members will not encourage a "loser" to join the team.

If it is a hygienist or chairside assistant being hired, I feel a member of the clinical staff should share in the selection process. When present staff participate in selecting a new employee, they tend to go out of their way to make the new person fit into the practice.

When possible, ask the top three applicants to work a day in the office before making the decision to hire. In some practices, this is the final step in the interview process. Applicants should be paid for their time. Dentists who utilize this procedure report it to be a very effective method for making the final selection.

Consider the way a person walks and talks. Slow walkers and talkers are usually slow workers. Dentistry is no place for people who move slowly.

Interviewing is a time-consuming activity. But when it is properly done, the rewards justify the investment. An interview is a form of test. It is advisable, therefore, to formulate in advance the questions to be asked.

The following comprehensive interview questions should prove helpful.* They were developed by Jill Janov and are from her booklet, "Hiring, Evaluating, and Firing: Critical Skills for Managers and Supervisors."

Job-Related Questions—General

Always ask open-ended questions, ones that don't indicate a desired answer.

1. Please describe your present responsibilities and duties.
2. How do you spend an average day?
3. How did you change the content of your job from when you assumed it to now?
4. Discuss some of the problems you've encountered on the job.
5. What do you consider your chief accomplishment in your present job?

To determine qualifications the applicant has in addition to work experience, ask:

1. How do you view the job for which you are applying?
2. What in your background particularly qualifies you to do the job?
3. If you were to obtain this job, in what areas could you contribute immediately?
4. In what ways have your education and training prepared you for the job?

---

*Reprinted by permission of Jill Janov., Wallingford Consulting Group, Wallingford, PA.

To probe for weaknesses:

1. What disappointments did you have in your previous job?
2. In what areas did you need help or guidance from your supervisor?
3. For what things has your supervisor praised you? Criticized you?
4. Of all the aspects of your last job, what did you like most? Least?

Job-Related Questions—Specific

1. How did you approach some of the problems on your previous job?
2. What were the results?
3. In your previous job, what percentage of your time was spent on [name a duty]?
4. What experience do you have with [name a specific duty or responsibility]?
5. What were some of the significant achievements of your work group as a result of your efforts?
6. What aspects of this position will be new to you? Which ones will require additional training, either on the job or technical, before you feel you can achieve proficiency?
7. Describe your strengths. Describe areas that need improvement, if any.

Questions that Uncover Personality Traits

MOTIVATION:
    Why did you select this type of career?
    What is it you seek in a job?
    What is your long-term career objective?
    What kind of position would you like to hold in five years? Ten?
    What do you want in your next job that you are not getting now?

STABILITY:
> What are your reasons for leaving your present job? Previous jobs?
> Why are you seeking a job now?
> What were your original career goals?
> Have they changed?
> What has been your greatest disappointment in terms of your career thus far? How did it change your thinking?

RESOURCEFULNESS:
> How did you change the scope of your previous job?
> What were some of the difficult problems encountered on the job? How did you solve them?
> What do you know about our practice?
> What do you know about the position you seek?
> What are the three most important assets you bring to this office?
> To whom did you go for counsel when you couldn't handle a job problem?
> What kind of problems did you bring to this person?

ABILITY TO WORK UNDER DIRECTION OR WITH OTHERS:
> Describe your doctor's supervisory methods. Evaluate them.
> For what things have you been complimented? Criticized?
> On what committees have you served?
> What did you contribute to each committee's work?
> In your previous jobs, how much of your work was done on your own? As part of a team?
> What qualities do you seek in a boss? What should your boss know about you to supervise you effectively?
> What should your team members know about you to work with you effectively?

FOR OFFICE ADMINISTRATORS:
> Describe how you manage others.
> How did you persuade the doctor to accept your new ideas?
> Describe your technique of getting a job done. What do you feel are the three key attributes of a successful manager?

Questions should assess only the knowledge, skills, abilities, and other work characteristics needed for entry-level performance or to learn the job, not those to be learned in training.

Questions should mirror the content of the job and fall into four basic categories: hypothetical, job knowledge, job simulation or job sample, and workover requirements.

Questions should assess requirements in proportion to their relative importance to adequate job performance.

Questions should be precise, complete, and unambiguous to avoid the need for clarification that would disrupt standardization and introduce potential bias.

All questions on the application-for-employment form should comply with the state and federal laws governing the hiring process. The federal law is the model and prevails unless state laws give more rights to the employee. Contact your state and local government offices for copies of the statutes and regulations governing business practices. They include information on the following:

Civil Rights Act
Equal Pay Act
Age Discrimination Act
National Labor Relations Act
Freedom of Information Act
Pregnancy Discrimination Act
Uniform Guidelines
Sexual Harassment Guidelines

After screening all applicants, there is merit in sending a letter of appreciation to each person who applied. One doctor I know mentions in the letter that if the applicant needs a personal dentist, he would be delighted to have his receptionist make an appointment. Believe it or not, the time he spends writing these letters has proven to be a practice-builder because many of the applicants have just moved to the area and have not selected a family dentist. Another dentist sends a long-stemmed rose to each applicant in the final interviewing process.

Training

The length of time required for training new staff members is determined by their previous experience and how easily they adapt to their new work environment.

If the office needs to dismiss a staff member for any reason, that person should never be asked to train his or her replacement. The doctor or another chairside assistant usually trains the incoming chairside personnel. Hygienists need the least amount of indoctrination because their duties are similar from office to office.

The office administrator normally trains the receptionist and other business auxiliaries. In smaller offices that lack administrators, the receptionists are trained by the doctor with the assistance of the clinical staff.

The weakest link in dental training is in the business area. For many years the business staff were "diamonds in the rough," polishing themselves through continuing education courses and dental publications. Now there are classes and audio and video programs especially developed for training business staff. These courses offer in-depth training and hands-on manuals. In addition, networking with other dental receptionists, bookkeepers, and office administrators is being increasingly utilized. Sharing ideas and experience through networking is extremely valuable.

When you are ready to make the job offer, make it in writing. The letter should state the salary, hours, position, title, main job descriptions, date of hire, and list of benefits. The probationary period should be clearly spelled out. Send two copies of the letter, asking the applicant to sign and return one copy for your personnel file. If it is not feasible to send an offer letter, have the applicant sign the job description portion of the application as part of the hiring process. This alleviates the possibility of future misunderstandings.

I recommend a 90-day trial period for every new employee. This introductory period allows the office and the employee adequate time to determine if the applicant is suited for the job. During this 90-day probationary period, the employee is ineligible for benefits. At the end of the trial period, the employee should receive an employee evaluation. (See sample forms in Figs. 1–1 and 1–2.) If the evaluation is favorable, the employee

```
Name _____ Date _____

                    Above              Below
        Excellent   Average   Average  Average   Poor
            1          2          3        4        5

1.  Patient Routine
    1 2 3 4 5  Getting patient into operatory
    1 2 3 4 5  Having chart where it's supposed to be
    1 2 3 4 5  Positioning chair
    1 2 3 4 5  Positioning patient in chair
    1 2 3 4 5  Nitrous oxide set correctly
    1 2 3 4 5  Nitrous nose-piece alcoholed off
    1 2 3 4 5  Having tray pre-set
    1 2 3 4 5  Reinforcing patient comfort
    1 2 3 4 5  Operatory clean before patient enters

2.  Treatment Procedures
    1 2 3 4 5  Instrument passing
    1 2 3 4 5  Use of air-water syringe
    1 2 3 4 5  Suctioning
    1 2 3 4 5  Being prepared for next step
    1 2 3 4 5  Quickness with amalgam
    1 2 3 4 5  Cementation
    1 2 3 4 5  Removal of cement
    1 2 3 4 5  Impressions
    1 2 3 4 5  Temporary crowns

3.  Emergencies
    1 2 3 4 5  Ability to handle efficiently
    1 2 3 4 5  Attitude toward

4.  Supplies
    1 2 3 4 5  Keeping supplies on hand
    1 2 3 4 5  Keeping supplies in operatory
    1 2 3 4 5  Ordering efficiently
    1 2 3 4 5  Inventory control

5.  Radiography
    1 2 3 4 5  Bite wings
    1 2 3 4 5  Periapicals
    1 2 3 4 5  Panoramics
    1 2 3 4 5  X-rays of root canals
    1 2 3 4 5  Paralleling technique
    1 2 3 4 5  Bisecting angle technique

6.  Patient Acceptance
    1 2 3 4 5  Patients seem to like
    1 2 3 4 5  Ability to converse with patients
    1 2 3 4 5  Ability to discuss dentistry

7.  Problem Solving
    1 2 3 4 5  Ability to handle equipment breakdown
    1 2 3 4 5  Ability to handle front office (phone, scheduling, etc.)
    1 2 3 4 5  Ability to handle patient problems (complaints, etc.)

8.  Staff Meetings
    1 2 3 4 5  Participation
    1 2 3 4 5  Ability to lead a meeting
    1 2 3 4 5  Ability to critique Doctor, staff members
    1 2 3 4 5  Ability to take constructive criticism
    1 2 3 4 5  Interest shown at staff meetings

9.  Attendance
    1 2 3 4 5  Attendance record
    1 2 3 4 5  When misses has a good excuse
    1 2 3 4 5  Punctuality
```

Fig. 1-1 Job review

```
10.  Appearance
     1 2 3 4 5   Hair
     1 2 3 4 5   Nails
     1 2 3 4 5   Clothes
     1 2 3 4 5   Weight
     1 2 3 4 5   Respiration
     1 2 3 4 5   Heart rate
     1 2 3 4 5   Health
     1 2 3 4 5   Overall appearance

11.  Attitude
     1 2 3 4 5   Toward high class
     1 2 3 4 5   Toward middle class
     1 2 3 4 5   Toward low class
     1 2 3 4 5   Toward toothaches
     1 2 3 4 5   Toward emergencies at end of day
     1 2 3 4 5   Personal attitude at 8:00 a.m.
     1 2 3 4 5   Personal attitude at 5:00 p.m.
     1 2 3 4 5   Toward staff members leaving early
     1 2 3 4 5   Toward Doctor leaving early

12.  Telephone
     1 2 3 4 5   Answering
     1 2 3 4 5   Ability to answer questions
     1 2 3 4 5   Personal calls don't interfere with work

13.  Continuing Education
     1 2 3 4 5   Reads dental magazines
     1 2 3 4 5   Attends meetings

14.  Free Time
     1 2 3 4 5   Finds things to do

15.  Problems (Please List)

16.  Overall Rating  1 2 3 4 5

17.  Salary:          Expect a raise?
     Satisfied?       If so, how much?
```

Fig. 1-1   *(Cont'd.)*

is placed on permanent status and furnished with a list of benefits.

Termination during the 90-day probationary period is indicated if the applicant does not perform satisfactorily or if he or she has not made significant progress after sufficient training. Such probationary terminations can be done without advance notice. It is important to select applicants with care because employee failures are very costly in terms of lost training time and production.

Every dental office should prepare a procedures manual that addresses everything from how to answer the telephone to how to dismiss a patient. Well-organized offices have staff members write out their duties in sufficient detail for a "fill-in staffer" to read through the appropriate passages and be able to function with little assistance from other staff members. Ideally, the procedures manual should be kept simple and up-to-date.

Ongoing training time needs to be scheduled each month for the dental staff. Such sessions may examine new materials and techniques, discuss seminars attended, or may be directed toward perfecting certain clinical or business skills.

Many dental offices set aside four hours per month for staff training and meetings. Keeping the lines of communication open and participating in training sessions pays high dividends. Such time expenditures are actually practice investments—some of the best investments that can be made.

I recommend that staff members take turns conducting training sessions. By so doing, special knowledge may be

EMPLOYEE'S NAME		POSITION TITLE			DATE OF REVIEW	
EMPLOYEE'S DEPARTMENT OR SECTION		IMMEDIATE SUPERVISOR			DATE EMPLOYED	
BEGINNING SALARY	PRESENT SALARY	AMOUNT OF LAST INCREASE	DATE OF LAST INCREASE	PROPOSED INCREASE	EFFECTIVE DATE	

PURPOSE OF THIS REVIEW

☐ COMPLETION OF PROBATIONARY EMPLOYMENT PERIOD (90 DAYS)   ☐ FIRST PERFORMANCE REVIEW OF THE YEAR
☐ SECOND PERFORMANCE REVIEW OF THE YEAR   ☐ ANNUAL SALARY REVIEW   ☐ PROMOTION   ☐ TRANSFER
☐ MARGINAL PERFORMANCE REVIEW   ☐ DISCIPLINARY REVIEW   ☐ TERMINATION

FACTORS	LOWEST ————————————————————————→ HIGHEST				
	1	2	3	4	5
PROMPTNESS Consider arrival at place of employment on time.	Seldom on time. ☐	Often tardy. Requires frequent warning. ☐	Occasionally late, but is conscientious about being at work. ☐	Has better record than average ☐	Never tardy without justifiable excuse. ☐
ABILITY TO LEARN Consider ability to understand and retain.	Very limited. ☐	Requires repeated instructions. ☐	Learns reasonably well. ☐	Rapidly understands and retains. ☐	Unusual capacity. ☐
POSITION KNOWLEDGE Consider the employee's knowledge of the job.	Knows only minimum for operating. ☐	Satisfied to limit knowledge to what is taught. ☐	Has the knowledge of the average worker on the job. ☐	Has knowledge required for success on job. ☐	Thorough knowledge of job and its function. ☐
INITIATIVE Consider originality and resourcefulness.	Lacking. ☐	Routine worker. ☐	Occasionally shows initiative. ☐	Better than average. ☐	Outstanding. ☐
JUDGMENT Consider ability to evaluate situations and make sound decisions.	Poor. ☐	Not always reliable. ☐	Good in most matters. ☐	Reliable. ☐	Decisions most logical and well founded. ☐
DEPENDABILITY Consider amount of supervision required and application to work.	Unreliable and inattentive. ☐	Needs frequent supervision. ☐	Generally reliable and attentive to work. Follows instructions carefully. ☐	Very reliable and conscientious, needs little supervision. ☐	Extremely reliable and industrious. ☐

Fig. 1–2 Employee evaluation record

FACTORS	LOWEST ──────────────────────────► HIGHEST				
	1	2	3	4	5
COOPERATION Consider cooperation with associates and supervisors.	Entirely uncooperative. ☐	Reluctant to cooperative. ☐	Adequately cooperative. ☐	Very Cooperative. ☐	Unusually cooperative. ☐
ATTITUDE TOWARD JOB Consider interest and enthusiasm.	Dislikes work. ☐	Shows little or no interest. ☐	Passive acceptance; rarely shows enthusiasm. ☐	Shows interest; enthusiasm is not sustained. ☐	Shows intense enthusiasm and interest in all work. ☐
QUANTITY OF WORK Consider the volume of work produced consistently.	Unsatisfactory output. ☐	Limited. Does just enough to get by. ☐	Average output. ☐	Above average producer. ☐	Exceptional output. ☐
QUALITY OF WORK Consider accuracy and neatness.	Very poor. ☐	Not entirely acceptable. ☐	Acceptable accuracy and neatness. ☐	Very neat and accurate. ☐	Exceptionally neat and accurate. ☐
SPEED Consider the rate at which the employee works.	Slow. ☐	Moderate. ☐	Average. ☐	Rapid. ☐	Exceptional. ☐

MAJOR STRENGTHS	MAJOR WEAKNESSES

SINCE EMPLOYEE'S LAST REVIEW, EMPLOYEE HAS
☐ IMPROVED ☐ MADE LITTLE OR NO CHANGE ☐ REGRESSED

WHAT IS YOUR OVERALL OPINION OF THIS EMPLOYEE
☐ UNSATISFACTORY ☐ POOR ☐ FAIR ☐ GOOD ☐ VERY GOOD ☐ OUTSTANDING

HAS THIS REVIEW BEEN DISCUSSED WITH EMPLOYEE?
☐ YES ☐ NO IF YES, ENTER DATE HERE

COMMENTS

RECOMMEND INCREASE ☐ YES ☐ NO	SUPERVISOR'S SIGNATURE	DATE

Fig. 1-2 Employee evaluation record *(Cont'd.)*

shared and staff members allowed to grow. Even the most timid staff members gain confidence when asked to demonstrate a procedure they perform well. The business staff person, for instance, might explain what she needs to improve patient flow at the front desk, e.g., cooperation from the entire team in completing routing slips, quick claims, or computer slips. The hygienist might demonstrate home care techniques so that any member of the staff can give such instructions. The assistant in charge of dental supplies might explain the inventory control system and tell how each staff person can assist in keeping inventory costs low. The doctor might demonstrate a new bonding technique or some other change in clinical dentistry. On occasion, the office could invite a doctor or a staff person from a specialty practice to enhance office knowledge in a particular area of expertise.

Training should be an ongoing experience and an integral part of every office's activities. Offices that learn together tend to stay together. They also are the offices that set goals, target dates, and reap the rewards of practice growth.

Wage Policies

Often staff members view dentistry as a dead-end job with no growth potential. Consequently, there is a high rate of turnover on many dental staffs. To build a stable dental staff, the wages and benefits offered must be comparable to other jobs in the immediate area.

Many dentists call my office and say, "Linda, I am getting ready to hire a new receptionist. "What is the average salary in my area?"

I inquire in return, "Do you want an average receptionist, Doctor?"

"Oh, no, I want above average."

If an office wants above-average people, it should be willing to pay above-average salaries. But to do that, the office must have above-average production.

I feel that staff salaries are the greatest investments a practice can make. I can always tell a lot about a practice when I meet the staff. Sharp offices hire sharp people, realizing they get what they pay for. One of my favorite lines about wage policies is

"If you pay peanuts, you get monkeys."

During consultations I talk to many staff members who feel they are grossly underpaid. I look at the percentage of the practice income that the office is paying for staff salaries. If the practice is paying above the average of 20 to 25 percent of the gross collected amount for staff salaries, then these staff members are not being underpaid. It would be more accurate to say that the office is underproducing for the number of people on staff.

When hiring a new employee, the office should pay that person less than the full agreed-upon beginning wage during the 90-day probationary period. After all, no matter how many years' experience this person has, the present staff will be spending many productive hours training the new auxiliary. If people are enthused about working in the practice, they'll realize that everyone pays dues to learn the ropes in a new business.

The worst sin an employer can make is to hire new employees at the same or higher salaries than senior staffers are being paid for the same job. The quickest way to lose the present staff is to commit this cardinal sin. Salaries should be confidential, but word can leak out and destroy practice morale.

I find that present staff members are much more receptive to training and accepting a new person if they feel they are appreciated for their past loyalty and dedication.

I emphasize praise and appreciation in all my seminars because it elevates self-esteem and morale. Overall morale, however, may be in real jeopardy three weeks or so after a new staff person joins because the old staff members get tired of hearing how great and cute the new employee is.

To make the transition smooth, praise the existing staff to the new employee with phrases like, "Karen has been my assistant for three years, Susan. She is excellent and practically reads my mind during a procedure." Such compliments to existing staff do two things: (1) they make Karen feel important and (2) they encourage Susan to become as effective as Karen.

Another example is this: "Ruth, rather than come to me with questions about the office, please go to Mary, our recep-tionist. She has been a valuable member of our team for five years and probably can give you a better answer than I can."

Such praising of existing staff is very important. Praising of the new staff person should be done privately until the other staffers feel she is pulling her weight. The existing staff will have difficulty accepting a new person who is getting all the praise when their last compliment was a year ago!

After the 90-day trial period, the new staff member should have an employee evaluation. Have the employee take copies of the evaluation home the night before the evaluation conference. She should grade herself and then compare her answers with those of the person conducting the evaluation—the doctor, office administrator, or other supervisor.

For instance, under "promptness," the new staff member may grade herself a 1 or 2, which is low or fair on a scale of 1 to 5. During the evaluation, the reviewing person should ask, "Ruth, what did you give yourself under promptness?" The new employee might say, "Well, I'm trying to be prompt, but I am not a morning person. I'm usually ten minutes late, so I gave myself a 2." The reviewer then might say, "Isn't that interesting? I gave you a 2 also." Self-evaluation is good because recognizing our faults takes us halfway to solving them.

The doctor or reviewing person should never mention salary at an evaluation conference. The employee is thinking, "How much am I going to get?" The reviewer is thinking, "How much does she expect?" The answers could be affected by this anticipation.

I recommend a merit increase review 30 days after the evaluation. Raises should be merit pay based on that person's worth to the practice. I suggest basing the amount of the merit pay on four things:

1. The staff person's attitude.
2. The evaluation weak areas that have been improved during the past 30 days.
3. The scope of responsibility since hiring or the last merit raise.
4. The growth of the practice since the last raise.

Existing staff should have an employee evaluation once a year in their anniversary month, with a merit increase review 30 days after their hiring anniversary date. If the total staff salary exceeds the 25 percent range, there can be no merit increases until production increases.

Staff members who have good attitudes enjoy evaluations and believe in merit pay. Those who are less than fully committed resent being evaluated and often feel they deserve more than is being offered.

Incentive bonuses are extra pay for extra effort and never take the place of annual merit increases. Incentives add fun and excitement to attaining goals. They are examined in the next chapter.

Many dentists ask how much of a raise is fair. If the practice isn't growing, neither can salaries. I am often asked, "When does a particular salary peak?" My response is, "When the practice stops growing—hopefully, never."

A simple formula for awarding raises is this: If staff salaries are 20–25 percent of the gross, take 10 percent of the office's increase in collections from one year to the next and divide that 10 percent among all staff (not necessarily evenly, but according to responsibility levels and worth to the practice as determined by the doctor and/or office administrator).

Example:

This year's collections	$434,000
Last year's collections	− 332,000
	$102,000
	× 0.10
	$ 10,200

$10,200 divided by 12 months =
  $850/month increase in salaries
Divide $850 by pay periods

Example:

Weekly is $850 divided by 4.3 = $198 (rounded)
Bimonthly is $850 divided by 2 = $425

Example:

Weekly ($198 divided)

7 years	office administrator	$ 40
2 years	receptionist	25
6 years	hygienist one	40
2 years	hygienist two	28
5 years	assistant one	30
2 years	assistant two	20
1 year	coordinating assistant	15
Total		$198

This is just an example. Merit raises depend on the scope of responsibility and worth to the practice of the individual staff members.

The services of a trained dental consultant may be indicated to assist with needs assessments for additional staff. The consultant also can offer suggestions of personality traits for particular jobs, outline job descriptions and delegation of duties, and assist with the interviewing and training processes.

This chapter should save time, money, and stress in assembling the winning office team. Advertising for staff, interviewing, training, and determining compensation policies are all integral parts of dental office success. Such measures should be viewed as the first steps in practice-building.

I advise graduating dental students regarding their first staff members: "If to attract the right first employee you must include her first year's salary in the office loan, do so. It makes all the difference in where the practice will be one, five, and ten years from now. It is false economy to try to save money when investing in staff."

Chapter 2

Motivating
the Staff

Motivation of dental staff comes easily for me because I was a dental staff member for many years. I can appreciate the frustrations dental personnel experience. In my case, my frustrations were compounded by a negative attitude.

Early in my career as an assistant, I felt my job was just a job. I lacked motivation and saw the dental environment as a negative work setting. Along with other staff members, I was frustrated by the lack of appreciation we experienced. I have since learned that in order to feel appreciation, one must give it. I didn't appreciate my dental bosses. In fact, if they asked me to go to a seminar, my first thought was, "Are we going to get paid for that evening or Saturday?"

Today I realize that my job didn't become a career until I dropped my negative attitude. At age 32 I worked as an endo assistant and began feeling differently toward my patients. Many of them commented on how I made their visits more pleasant. The doctor complimented me on my ability to communicate with patients. About then, I began feeling good about my role as an assistant.

From 1976 to 1980 I had the privilege of working in a totally positive atmosphere for a very appreciative boss. All my previous dental bosses had been excellent dentists who treated their staffs well, but never before had I met a dentist who put the entire staff on a colleague level. In that office I watched average employees blossom and reach their full potential as auxiliaries.

I began to study moods and personalities and realized how they affect attitudes. If everyone in the office came to work in a good mood, we interacted well and even the patients commented on our happy, caring office. On the other hand, if one person was in a bad mood, it affected our team attitudes and had an adverse effect on production. Happy employees and employers are far more productive.

Reasons for Incentives

At that office we always set goals, usually reached them, and then shared in rewards of extra money, paid trips, or gifts. Such activities created fun within the office.

Several years after I began giving seminars, I was asked to write an article on motivation. I remembered back to my years as an average, unmotivated employee and what had happened in my personal life and career after I changed.

In the article I spoke of the three *R*s of motivation—the fundamental motivating factors for all human behavior:

Responsibility
Recognition
Rewards

We all need responsibility: a reason to get up in the morning, to go to work, to perform. Responsibility gives us a sense of being and purpose. With responsibility, we also need recognition. Without recognition in the form of praise and appreciation, we give less than our best to a job.

Rewards are extra incentives over and above our regular pay. Staff who feel there's "something in it for me" are far more excited about contributing to practice growth. I have witnessed practices that doubled when employee attitudes became "we" rather than "me." Progress can be defined as everyone in the office pulling in the same direction at the same time. Incentives that are well designed and that originate in a desire to share can definitely enhance a dental practice.

Destructive Incentives

Many dentists, with good reason, shy away from incentive bonus plans. This is because some incentive plans create more problems than motivation. The most harmful incentive plan is one that has different goals and rewards for different staff members. This type of plan creates staff competition and jealousy, a fertile soil for intraoffice conflict.

A poorly conceived incentive plan is illustrated by a dentist who goes to the staff person responsible for collections and says, "Peggy, if you can collect over 95 percent of the fees each month, you will receive a $100 bonus." Then he goes to his clinical staff and says, "Okay, assistants and hygienists, if you can help me produce a certain amount each month, you will each get $100."

It takes two or more weeks for an insurance check to arrive. Therefore, if Peggy puts a large insurance case on the appointment book toward the end of the month, her collections might not be over 95 percent and she will lose her bonus. The clinical staff, on the other hand, will get a bonus because their results are measured immediately. As a consequence, Peggy may be tempted to appoint that large insurance case after the first of next month. Production begins with the telephone, appointment book, and pencil.

Another incentive plan that doesn't work very well is one based on monthly collections. Such a plan places too much pressure on the one or two people in the office responsible for collections. The clinical staff have very little control over payment arrangements and collections of past due accounts. A dental office can only be as successful as the money collected. But if the staff members are to share in the bonus, they also should share in the responsibility of income.

A doctor at one of my seminars told me about an incentive plan he had designed. He made this prediction: "Linda, I just know you are going to talk about my incentive plan at all your seminars." And I do. This doctor said to his receptionist of four years, "Barbara, we have a severe collections problem—only 79 percent has been collected." To get Barbara more enthused about working on the past-due accounts, he said, "Beginning the first of next month, I want you to work on the past-due accounts at home. You may keep 20 percent of anything you collect that is over 120 days old." Guess what this ingenious receptionist did? She let every account in the office go over 120 days so she could get the 20 percent. In fact, she stopped sending statements. Incentives have been known to backfire, and this was one that did.

Another incentive plan that can create a problem is one based on a monthly figure. Let us say the office is currently producing $30,000 per month. The doctor tells the staff that if they can produce $33,000 per month, they will all get a nice check. As you know, some months are high, others are not: dentistry is "seasonal" in many offices. And what if the doctor decides to take his or her spouse on a vacation to Mexico? About midmonth, the staff realizes the week off will defeat the possibility of reaching the month's goal. Since the bonus is impossible, there is the obvious temptation to save all the big cases until the following month.

Incentives that Work

If you want an incentive to work, it has to be fair to everyone. Fair also means that the goals must be realistic.

I believe in a graduated incentive plan, one that does not require a full-time bookkeeper to keep score. Simplicity and fairness are the basis for all our systems. I believe in the KISS concept ("Keep It Simple, Sweetie").

If the incentive is based on a daily average, the staff is continually aware of the goal. Basing the goal on such an average is fair. If the doctor takes a week off, the goal is not altered. Staff who perform behind the scenes practice-building activities when the doctor is out know they are producing even though their work is not directly with patients. The result of these efforts shows up later in the production figures.

Both production and collections figures should be incorporated into an incentive plan. To determine a fair first goal, add together the last three months' production and collections, then divide by two. Now count the number of days the office saw patients in these three months. Divide the number of days (which may end with 0.5 for a half day) into the total of the production and collection divided by two. The resulting number is a mean average per day. Then add $100 per day per doctor to the daily mean as a realistic first goal.

If the goal is reached the next month, all full-time staff receive $50 (minus taxes).* All part-time staff are prorated (3 days per week = $30, etc.). After reaching or exceeding the goal for three consecutive months, set a new goal and a new reward for the coming month by adding the three mean averages attained for the past three months, dividing by three, and then adding $100 per day to the resultant number. Now the reward should be $75 for each full-time staff person.

An example of this system follows. When the average of the past three months' production and collections is divided by 2 and then divided again by the number of days worked, the past three months, the result is $1,008. As a first goal in a one-doctor office, add $100 to that figure to make $1,108 per day. Let's presume that the mean average in the first month is $1,127, a bonus month; the second month is $1,154, another bonus month; and the third month is $1,205, a third bonus month in a row.

$1,127 + 1,154 + 1,205 = $3,486

$3,486 ÷ 3 = $1,162 + 100 = $1,262/day (second goal)

In the fourth month the office produces $1,283; in the fifth month someone on the staff is ill and production slips to $1,235 (below bonus level). In nonbonus months, staff members receive only their normal paychecks because bonuses are extra pay for extra results. Staff should not expect to achieve a bonus every single month, but 9 or 10 out of 12 is great. The fifth month is not a bonus month, so the sixth month becomes month one for the $1,262 goal. If a month is missed, the goal remains the same until it has been attained for three consecutive months. Once that has happened, new goals and new rewards are established.

If an office has two doctors and one is less productive than the other, prorate the daily average. Example, Dr. A is off on Friday, leaving Dr. B (the new associate) alone with a skeleton

---

*Bonus checks are separate and go on the payroll record as extra income. Taxes must be withheld.

staff. Dr. B's daily average is 25 percent of the two-doctor, two-hygienest production. For bonus purposes, count Fridays as one-fourth of a day.

Being made aware of bonus status on a daily basis tends to produce extra efforts. In one office the bookkeeper posts a number daily on the staff lounge refrigerator door. It might be, for instance, −$42, which means the office is $42 per day short of reaching its goal for the month. Let's keep those chairs filled and get all the emergencies in cheerfully. If the refrigerator door says +$23, it means the office is $23 per day above the daily goal. Let's keep going!

Incentives make working as a team fun. Satisfaction similar to reaching our own goals results from helping others reach theirs. Remember that people without goals are usually those who feel "Good enough is OK" or "We should be motivated without incentive." Money, useful as it is, is not a totally satisfactory motivator. But sharing goal attainment with others while delivering quality care to patients makes for a wonderful combination.

Tangible Fringe Benefits

It's been said that money is not important; it's just second in line to oxygen. Perhaps, but cash incentives are not the only motivating factors for the dental team. Other motivators include fringe benefits such as the following:

Time off with pay

Personal time to take care of errands and family needs is great while receiving the same paycheck amount. One doctor I know tells the staff on their final interview, "I pay my staff for 40 hours per week. If we get the job done in 36 hours, the staff takes Friday afternoons off with pay." This "free" afternoon compensates for any overtime they may have put in at lunch or quitting times. However, if his office has a big project such as purging patient records or redoing the filing system, then the Friday afternoon is withdrawn with three weeks' notice. This doctor also allows his staff to rotate days off with pay while he attends continuing education courses.

Uniform allowances

Many offices provide the staff with a uniform allowance. This is a separate, tax-free check that usually is issued monthly. Amounts vary from $10 to $40. The Internal Revenue Service frowns on anything over $50. For tax purposes, staff members who receive a uniform allowance must keep receipts for their business-related purchases. If they are audited and cannot show receipts equal to their annual benefit, the difference is taxable as additional gross income.

Well bonus

Buying back unused sick days at full pay is another benefit offered in many offices. Some offices pay an additional bonus of $100 or so to staff members who have not used any sick days during the year. These well bonuses are paid during the staff member's anniversary month for the year just ended. A well bonus is income and is taxable like other salary.

Free dentistry

Many offices offer free dentistry to staff members after one year of service. Often a 20 to 25 percent fee reduction also is offered to the staff member's immediate family. It obviously is imperative for staff members to maintain their teeth in excellent repair. Some offices designate one day per quarter as Staff Day. On that day everyone in the office (including the doctor) has his or her teeth cleaned and restored.

Continuing education

This fringe benefit should be considered by every dental office. Staff members who share learning experiences work together better and are more interested in promoting growth of the practice. Those who view continuing education as an infringement on their time are working at jobs, not careers. Worthwhile courses that educate and motivate are investments that pay for themselves many times over.

Insurance or medical reimbursements

Medical plans can be the most costly fringe benefit a practice can offer. And sometimes they're not even appreciated.

Staff members often complain their medical insurance deductions are so high that it's like having no benefit at all. If the office selects a plan with a low deductible, the premiums can be very high indeed.

Some offices offer direct reimbursement plans to their staff members. One such plan pays $100 for each day worked per week to full-time and part-time staff members.

Example:

5 days per week = $500 per year maximum

3 days per week = $300 per year maximum

1 day per week = $100 per year maximum

Staff members bring receipts for prescriptions and medical and dental treatments. They are directly reimbursed up to the amount of their yearly maximum. Direct reimbursement plans are being well received by staff members. They have the obvious advantages of eliminating insurance premiums, deductions from the payroll, and related paperwork requirements.

Health spa memberships

Members of the dental team should be physically fit. Spa memberships encourage fitness and are appreciated by most staff members. In some offices staff members go to the spa a couple of times a week during extended lunch periods. A workout, shower, and light lunch bring staff back to the office supercharged and ready for a productive afternoon.

Association membership dues

Only a small percentage of dental staff members belong to professional associations. I urge dental offices to encourage such memberships by offering to pay the dues. The networking and exchange of ideas that occurs at association meetings is valuable.

Intangible Fringe Benefits

Besides special tangible fringe benefits, employees appreciate the following intangible benefits.

Personal business cards

Having personal business cards can make staff members feel important and be a practice-builder as well. All staff members should be furnished with business cards that include their name and title along with the doctor's (or office's) name, address, and telephone number.

Nameplates on door

Staff members feel especially important if their nameplates are on the door leading from the reception room to the treatment rooms. Such nameplates also make favorable impressions on patients (if the staff is important, so are the patients). Having a new staff person's nameplate engraved and in position on the first day of work is a warm welcome to the office.

Personal photographs

Everyone has a favorite photo of a parent, spouse, child, niece, nephew, or pet. Having such photographs on display personalizes the office and helps patients feel more relaxed through the realization that the doctors and staff are real people. Encouraging staff to display personal photos makes them feel they're recognized as people and not simply as employees.

Titles

Titles bring status and prestige. Titles look good on business cards, stationery, and door plates. Activities that consume a third or more of our lives deserve titles.

I have never cared for the title "office manager." That title has caused dissention among staff members who resent being "managed" by someone they look upon as a co-worker. The title "office administrator" sounds more professional and meets better acceptance. Team players are more receptive to being administered to than managed.

The title "receptionist" is not entirely satisfactory to encompass all the duties a front desk person performs. Most dental receptionists are appointment book engineers, official hostesses, bill-payers, bankers, secretaries, bookkeepers, payroll clerks, insurance clerks, and sometimes babysitters and cab-callers as well. The title "administrative assistant" or "business assistant" sometimes better describes the position.

Dental assistants should use their full title on cards, stationery, and other printed items. Some examples of the titles encountered include certified dental assistant, registered dental assistant, expanded duty assistant, and dental aide. Some offices have coordinating dental assistants who are referred to as "rovers." While admittedly descriptive, that particular title might look better in a veterinarian's office than a dentist's.

Hygienists also should use their full title on cards and stationery. Degrees are appropriately added by hygienists who hold them.

Surprises Are Fun

Some dentists enjoy giving surprise bonus incentives that add zest and appreciation to a routine practice. One dentist in Florida has a Staff Appreciation Fun Day each December. He makes reservations at a fabulous restaurant for lunch. The day before Fun Day, he tells his staff to report to work at 10 A.M. in casual attire. After a short staff meeting, they go to lunch from about 11 A.M. to 2 P.M. Then he drives them to a shopping mall, hands them each a $100 bill, and says, "Meet me here at 4 P.M. with your change!" The dentist says these have been some of the greatest days of his life.

At one of our three-day institute classes for dental business staff, an attendee from Tennessee said, "I work for the greatest dentist in the world. Two years ago he started sending his staff of six on an expense-paid cruise when he takes his family on vacation!" Needless to say, everyone in the class agreed when she said she worked for the world's greatest dentist. As a matter of fact, some of them took his name and telephone number on the chance he might have a staff vacancy!

In my experience, dental offices with well-designed incentive plans produce 30 to 40 percent more than those without. In the absence of motivating factors in the practice, there is a similar lack of patient motivation. Unfortunately, too many dentists never learn the secret of sharing the growth of their practices with those who have made it happen. Perhaps that's why so few dental practices ever reach their full potential.

Many dentists use the excuse, "I don't want my patients to feel rushed or mistreated by overly enthusiastic staff." The truth, however, is that staff who feel appreciated go out of their way to render quality care. They know how important the extra mile is to the practice. Remember, in order to give love, you must feel love, and in order to give respect and trust, you must feel respect and trust. Going back to basics, staff motivation is simply "Do unto others as you would have them do unto you"—the Golden Rule for the golden practice.

Chapter 3

Communications with Each Other

The importance of strong intraoffice communication is outlined in this chapter. Many dental offices stay so busy interpreting patients' communication needs, they often overlook the team's communication needs.

Staff meetings that allow everyone to participate can lead to the winning team attitude—an absolute necessity if the office is to move up from one production level to another. People (both staff members and doctors) must feel appreciated, goals must be set and reevaluated, and communication must be open.

Staff meetings that motivate rather than alienate open the doors to real communication and create excitement. They are a "turn-on"!

Meetings that Motivate

Communication is probably the most important ingredient in a successful dental practice because it is *the* basis for organization, motivation, and appreciation. Without good communication, nothing can happen.

There is no better vehicle for improving intraoffice communication than a staff meeting. Open and informative staff meetings enhance the office atmosphere, lead to a more organized practice, and cause staff members to become self-motivated and committed.

Motivating others to higher levels of performance is a task that is difficult at best and often seems impossible. On the other hand, if an atmosphere can be created that fosters self-motivation, then goals—both individual and group—start being attained. Staff meetings are crucial to the development of such an atmosphere. When held for the right reasons and properly conducted, staff meetings can be the most productive portion of the week or month.

Many offices avoid staff meetings because they are actually gripe sessions and tend to make everyone feel worse instead of better. In too many offices, staff meetings are called only when the doctor has complaints about the staff that can no longer be be contained. In such instances attendees view staff meetings as disagreeable and threatening. Meetings of this type can be very destructive because criticism abounds. Criticism in front of others is detrimental to the criticized person's self-esteem. At such times, communication cannot exist. Staff meetings should be a time to discuss practice problems, not people problems.

Staff meetings should always be planned. They are best scheduled for the first hour or two of the practice day, at least once a month, and at a specific time. It is always desirable to have staff meetings when everyone is fresh and rested. Some offices have their meetings weekly, others bimonthly, and there are a few who have brief meetings at the start of every day. Incoming calls should be handled as if the staff were attending an off-site seminar. Interruptions undermine the effectiveness of the staff meeting. Presuming there's a planned agenda, the more frequent the meetings, the greater the communication possibilities. In the absence of an agenda, a staff meeting may be seen as an annoyance and a waste of time.

If once-a-month staff meetings are productive, the more casual, coffee-break meetings may be too short to meet the communication needs of the office. In some offices, however, short meetings are very effective. One of my favorite offices routinely schedules a 15-minute coffee-break meeting every morning sometime between 9 and 11 A.M. On the appointment book, this time is reserved for "Mr. Rodney." For that particular office (which is one of the most relaxed, appreciative, and productive offices I have ever visited), these brief but regular meetings are an important part of their success.

Staff meetings should be held early in the month, preferably the first Tuesday, Wednesday, Thursday, or Friday. (Monday mornings are usually too hectic with incoming phone calls.) Meetings that are scheduled for the first week of the month allow the office to evaluate progress and to set new goals before the month is far along. If new goals are established mid-month or later, there can be little enthusiasm for reaching them. Staff meetings always should be held on office time, not on staff time. The late Bob Barkley said, "If you pay staff to think, they think so much better."

Each staff member should have a turn at conducting the staff meetings. This gives everyone in the office a sense of importance. One month the hygienist may be in charge and the next month someone from the business staff or an assistant or the doctor. Rotating responsibility tends to make everyone feel equally important. One of the best staff meetings I ever attended was conducted by a 21-year-old dental assistant.

If the doctor has misgivings about losing a couple of hours of production for a staff meeting, it should be noted that improving intraoffice communication may well be the most productive time of the entire month.

By nature, dental offices involve small numbers of people working closely together in situations that often are intense. As a by-product of this environment, staff and doctor become "family," and suggestions for improvements may never be brought into the open for fear of stepping on someone's toes. To alleviate this problem, I recommend placing a locked suggestion box in the lab.

All staff members and doctor(s) are asked to anonymously type at least two suggestions per month and place them in the box. The suggestions should be positive ideas that will save time and money or reduce stress and tension. It is important that each team member be required to offer at least two ideas. Of course, more are welcome, but participation is the first requisite of any team.

On the last day of the month, the doctor unlocks the suggestion box, puts all the ideas into an envelope, and gives them to the person in charge of the next monthly staff meeting. Once the ideas are read at the staff meeting, the staff may vote on the best suggestion of the month. I recommend $20 be given for the winning suggestion. If two or more staff members have submitted the same idea, then the reward should be split accordingly. Not only are rewards an incentive to keep staff and doctors constantly looking for ways to improve the practice, they also add fun to the staff meeting.

Monthly progress reports on different aspects of the practice should be presented at staff meetings by those responsible in the various areas. As I often say to audiences of auxiliaries, "If you don't tell your doctors and co-workers what wonderful work you are doing, they may never know." This form of communication also lets the clinical staff understand the importance of the work of the business staff and vice versa. Personal progress reports urge staff members to do more. They become their own competition. They also become more aware of what other staff members are doing to build the practice, thus creating appreciation for them.

There are numerous reasons for giving monthly progress reports:

They give each team member an "outside the normal line of duty" responsibility and make him or her feel they contribute extras.

They make each staff member understand and appreciate the efforts of others.

They increase enthusiasm.

They let the doctor know what has been accomplished behind the scenes in the past month, thus improving staff-to-doctor communication.

They help doctors evaluate each staff member's contribution and provide a means of measurement in determining merit increases.

Staff meetings should be planned well in advance so everyone comes prepared to participate. Below are some suggested topics for staff meetings:

Last month's production.

Last month's collection.

Last month's percentage of collections (average good collections would be 95 to 98 percent).

The number of new patients last month (a healthy number is 25 to 40 per month per doctor, including emergencies).

The percentage of overhead expenses last month. Staff who know overhead figures feel more a part of the team than those who do not know. (The average general practice has a true overhead in the 60 to 70 percent range.)

The amount spent on supplies last month and the percentage. (Divide the total supply costs by the total amount collected for percentage. A "good" average is in the range of 5 to 7 percent.)

The number of patients the hygienist averaged per day last month, the number of "holes" in the schedule that were not filled, and the average number of dollars produced per day. (A productive hygienist generates between $300 and $375 per day, depending on the office's fee schedule.)

The number of patients who tried to break an appointment without at least 24 hours' notice. (See the appointment book control for tracking this figure.) The progress report should read, "Last month, 57 patients tried to change or break an appointment without proper notification. I was able to maintain 43." Talk about valuable! Such a person's worth is hard to measure.

The number of delinquent account calls made last month and the amount of dollars collected on bad debts.

The average dollars per day (add the total production and total collections and divide by the number of days patients are seen).

The incentive bonuses reached for the month and presentation of the appropriate checks.

The number of patients who reappointed after purging calls, as well as the number of patients who left the practice and their reasons for leaving.

New goals and target dates.

At the end of the staff meeting, the leader for the next month should be appointed. A staff meeting report should be typed and a copy given to each staff member (Fig. 3–1). In addition, an office copy should be filed for future reference.

Doctor: _____

Date: _____

Staff in attendance: _____

_____

_____

Conducted by: _____

Staff position: _____

Agenda:

_____

_____

_____

_____

Reports:

Number of new patients the previous month: _____

Number of patients changing or breaking an appointment: _____

Number you were able to keep on the book at that time: _____

Last month's production: _____

Last month's collections: _____

Percentage of collections: _____

Number of delinquent account calls made: _____

Amount collected as a result of those calls: _____

Average dollars/day produced and collected divided by 2: _____

Goal for average dollars per day: _____

Incentive bonus amount received: _____

Fig. 3–1 Sample staff meeting report

Amount of money spent on supplies: —————————————————

Percentage of overhead for the month: —————————————

Number of purged telephone calls made: —————————————

Number appointed: —————————————————————————————

Number that have left the practice: —————————————————

Reasons for leaving: —————————————————————————————

———

———

New Ideas:

———

———

———

———

Goals:

Production: ————————————————————————————————————

Collections: ————————————————————————————————————

Number of new patients: —————————————————————————

Attitudes: —————————————————————————————————————

Our biggest accomplishment as a team last month was ——————

———

———

Our goal to strive for this month will be ————————————————

———

———

Fig. 3–1   Sample staff meeting report *(Cont'd.)*

A positive office atmosphere and good staff morale are not accidents. Staff meetings that motivate, not alienate, are a means to achieve these ends.

Appreciation and Trust Are Contagious

Many dentists express the feeling that their staffs do not appreciate them. There's a reason for that. Before the staff members can show appreciation, they must feel appreciation. Too often that fails to happen.

Other dentists say, "I should do away with these staff benefits such as profit-sharing and paid personal days." In defense of the staff on this valid complaint, more than half the auxiliaries I meet do not understand their benefits package. This is why benefits, right along with goals and duties, should be outlined in an office manual and made a part of every staff member's initial indoctrination.

Get the art of appreciation going in the practice today. Remember, you can't show it until you feel it. Start complimenting each other and the patients. Start looking for the positive rather than the negative. You will find exactly what you look for in a job, in your work, and even in your play. Have you ever known someone going to Las Vegas who said, "I'm only taking what I can afford to lose"? Guess what. They lost—usually the precise amount they'd planned. Their subconscious mind had expected to lose, and they did. We make prophecies, and then we fulfill them. The trick is to make positive prophecies rather than negative ones. You may call such things game-playing, but they work.

Never criticize a staff member in front of others. If a reprimand is necessary, do it in private. If the office has particularly slow workers (or 70-percenters, as we call them), start noticing the right things they do. Compliment them, and then watch the improvement. Behavior that is appreciated is repeated. Pretty soon these employees will be jumping through hoops to please those who praise them. After a while the entire office atmosphere will begin to improve. This feeling of appreciation really is contagious. Try it; you'll like it!

Some practitioners are hesitant about sharing the office collection/production/expense figures. In most instances sharing such information is much more productive than not sharing it. Trust breeds loyalty. I often ask employers, "How would you like to be on a football team and play your heart out but never know the score?" If you don't know what is happening, how can you know about what needs to happen? If staff members don't know a good day from a bad day, the job becomes just a job: "Give me my paycheck and let me out of here."

While consulting, I interview hundreds of staff members. In nonsharing offices, staff members say, "Our boss doesn't trust us" or "Only his bookkeeper or wife knows those figures." In sharp, progressive offices, by contrast, staff members are aware of both goals and current status. Of course, there are some numbers that are not shared, such as who takes what home in the way of a paycheck.

All big businesses share figures with employees in annual reports. If staff members are expected to have a personal interest in the practice, then information needs to be shared with all. If staff members are expected to think *our* patients and *our* office, trust is a necessary prerequisite.

A recent study shows that companies that communicate company goals and policies to their employees have a low turnover and a high yield level of loyalty from their people. Employees who feel they are needed, who know their contribution is important, and who are involved in what happens in the company are loyal and hardworking. If leadership has "secrets" from the employees, cooperation is minimal.

Loyalty and How It Affects Production

Loyalty means working hard with an attitude of "What can I do for my patients, doctor, and co-workers?" rather than "What can this practice do for me?"

Loyalty, remember, comes from trust. If employees feel trusted, they become loyal. Loyalty is working until the last patient is cared for, realizing the dental office is not a 9-to-5 job, never talking about patients with anyone other than staff, coming to work when you would rather not, and being supportive of the dentist, staff, and dentistry in all contacts with others.

Productivity increases in dental offices when staff members and doctors become loyal. Loyalty creates a happy working environment. Patients make referrals to happy offices.

In dental offices where good interpersonal relationships exist, patients feel more secure. Good relationships are the result of mutual appreciation, trust, and loyalty. Patients sense these attitudes, feel more secure themselves, and are more confident in making recommendations to others.

Communication with co-workers fails most often when we are unsure of goals, do not listen to each other's needs, and don't appreciate the contributions of the other members of the team. Communication requires participation, commitment, and enthusiasm. One of the secrets of those who find their careers exciting is their involvement. As an office administrator once said to me, "I thought I needed to change jobs. But I now realize that what I really needed to change was *me*."

Chapter 4

Communications with Patients

The office atmosphere can change markedly for the patients and dental team if everyone in the office makes a concerted effort to improve communications from the initial telephone contact to completion. In a "dynamicized" practice—one that believes in treating patients specially—dramatic improvements occur in both attitude and production level when effective communications begin to take place.

Eight Phases of the Patient's Visit

The most successful practices today share a common denominator: staff members skilled in public relations who know how to save their doctors many hours per week by communicating for them.

Fig. 4–1 shows the eight phases of communication that occur during a patient's visit. Seven of the eight are interactions solely between the patient and staff members. Obviously, good communication skills on the part of staff members are essential.

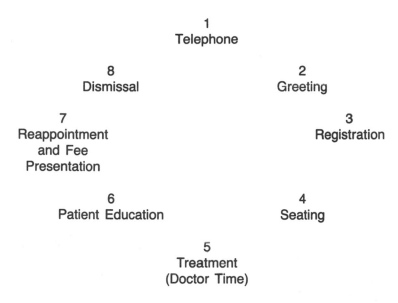

Fig. 4–1.   The eight phases of communication

Phase One: Telephone

Answering the telephone is the most important phase of all communication. The patient's initial impression of the office is formed during the first 30 seconds of the telephone contact. The person answering the telephone should sound enthusiastic and caring. "Dead wood" on the telephone has lost many potential new patients for dental practices.

The telephone is the initial point of contact for most new patients, and the atmosphere of a happy, caring doctor's office can be created immediately if the person answering has a smile in his or her voice. First impressions are lasting ones. You may never get a second chance to correct a "Hello" that was grumpy. In addition, patients who are sitting in the reception area are reassured and cheered by the sound of a pleasant voice. Every aspect of an environment has an effect.

If the receptionist cannot answer the telephone on the first few rings, the office is understaffed. This is a problem in many dental practices. Patients calling the office can only hear the ringing or busy signal. They cannot see a patient standing in front of the desk, being helped. However, the patient at the desk hears the telephone and understands that it must be answered.

When new patients get busy signals, they may forget to call back or, worse yet, look for another dentist who isn't so busy. A busy signal is one of the fastest ways to kill a practice. Putting a patient on "hold" is also a quick way to chill enthusiasm. Being placed on hold says very clearly that the caller is not important enough to rate immediate attention. Subsequent efforts to sound happy and caring tend to be dismissed by those who have been on hold too long.

Receptionists may have top-notch telephone skills, but these skills cannot be properly utilized if there is but one incoming telephone line. Most telephone companies will conduct peak load studies that monitor the number of busy signals your telephone line has per hour. If the average is more than two busy signals per hour, the office needs another incoming line. Remember, *busy people hate busy signals.* An investment in adequate equipment is insignificant compared to the new patients that may be lost by an office appearing to be too busy. A dental practice can only be as adequate as the telephone system.

Most dental offices should have no less than two incoming rotary lines and a third private line for outgoing calls and incoming personal calls. A competent telephone receptionist should be able to handle three lines in a professional manner. The first caller always has priority, so make the second answer brief—call back if you must. Never answer with, "Can you hold, please? [Click.]." To the first caller say, "Excuse me, Ms. Jones. My other line is ringing. I'll be right back." To the second caller say, "Good morning. Dr. Wood's office. This is Mary. I have another call. Can you hold for a few moments, or may I call you back?" Anytime someone is on hold, brevity is the byword.

Successful practices will get more than 400 new patients a year per doctor or 33 per month. That is a lot of "first impressions" to make. Why not make them good? The telephone is a wonderful marketing tool if used correctly. With a little effort, the entire tone of the dental experience gets off to a great start when patients are made to feel important. Investing in more telephone lines and learning to use them repays itself many times over. Answering the telephone with a cheerful and caring manner makes every patient feel special.

Receptionists always should answer the telephone by identifying the office and themselves: "Good morning. Dr. Wood's office. This is Mary." If the receptionist identifies the office only, the caller is speaking to an object (cold and unresponsive). By identifying themselves, receptionists have begun on a friendly, caring note with the caller. It is annoying for callers to have to ask, "Is this Betty, Joan, or Mary?" Even in a one-staff-member office, it is still good telephone manners for the answering person to identify herself.

One of the biggest telephone mistakes in a dental office is asking the caller, "Have you been a patient here before?" Even if the person answering the telephone is new to the practice, there is the risk of insulting patients of record by failing to recognize them. People love to feel important. The caller may be someone who completed a large treatment plan last month. If the receptionist is unfamiliar with the caller, ask, "How long has it been since your last appointment with the doctor?" By doing this, the risk of insulting either a new or former patient has been minimized.

If the caller is a new patient, the receptionist should find out if a routine office visit is needed or if there is a particular problem by asking, "Are you having an immediate problem?" Use of the words "pain" or "hurt" should be avoided, as they are negative words in dentistry. If the new patient indicates there is an immediate problem, the staff should be maximally responsive. Emergency patients become enthusiastic missionaries for dental practices.

Some offices regard emergencies as interruptions to their routine. Such offices could be missing as much as $30,000 to $80,000 a year by not welcoming emergencies. Emergency patients who are well treated will return, and they can be counted on for $1,000 per year in continued care and referrals. If you take good care of emergency patients, they will go back to their offices and tell everyone how great they were treated. That is how practices grow.

Some doctors and staff need to change their attitudes about an emergency. This involves a patient who needs attention now. Upon learning of an emergency, the receptionist should ask, "How soon can you be here?" This is soothing to the patient. The patient is being told that the office is willing to drop everything to attend to his or her need. If it is truly an emergency, the patient will be in as soon as possible. If he or she can't make it until after work, then you may presume this is not a true emergency and the patient can wait for a regular appointment.

This method differentiates the true emergencies from those of less urgency. It only takes a few minutes to seat, examine, and X-ray a patient. Two or three emergencies per day will not disrupt the schedule if the office is well equipped and staffed. (More about proper staffing in appointment book control.)

The receptionist should give directions to the office to all new patients, even if the office is easy to locate. She should ask these patients to arrive ten minutes before their scheduled appointment so there will be time to fill out the necessary forms.

During the patient's initial call, the receptionist also should ask, "Whom may we thank for referring you to our office?" This verbalizes the office philosophy "We *love* new patients." Even though the same questions may be asked on the patient information form, the receptionist should inquire about the referring party at the first contact.

A file with alphabetical patient cards makes it easy to keep track of referrals in noncomputerized offices. If the caller says, "My neighbor, Joan Black, referred me," Black's referral card should be pulled and the date and new patient's name written on it. The card should not be refiled until the referral has been acknowledged with a thank-you note or small gift.

The receptionist should say something nice about the referring party. For example, "Joan Black is one of my favorite patients—I always look forward to her visits" or "Joan Black refers such nice people to us." This is good public relations because the new patient probably will call Joan Black and tell her about the compliment. Joan Black will be apt to refer more patients to the office because she is held in such high regard there.

People love to be appreciated. It is a good idea to send handwritten, informal notes to each referring patient. If a patient is especially loyal and refers several new patients, the office may want to do something special. Flowers are nice for women; fruit baskets are appreciated by both sexes. For either men or women, lunch for two or theatre tickets are nice ways to say "thank you." Letting referring patients know they are appreciated is good for them and good for the practice.

Another question that should be asked during the new-patient telephone interview is "Do you have any dental insurance?" Third-party plans are increasingly common as more employers realize they must offer competitive benefit packages. If the caller has such coverage, then he or she must bring claim forms to the office.

Another consideration of telephone management is the amount of time that is spent on personal calls. Personal calls can disrupt the efficiency of any office. If the receptionist spends a lot of time answering calls for the doctor and staff about their personal business, then how she is being utilized must be evaluated. It is all well and good for the doctor to be involved in outside activities such as social and civic groups. But these activities must not interfere with the dental practice. The patient in the chair deserves everyone's undivided attention.

In a well-organized practice, the administrative assistant has the authority to "cluster" the doctor's incoming calls, except for emergencies. The doctor should give the receptionist a short list of those persons and situations for which he will take chairside interruptions. These may include family emergencies, other doctors, and long-distance calls. The receptionist should never announce the calls chairside; patients will feel they are less than top priority.

Instead, the receptionists should write notes or use a light signaling system for those few interruptions that require the doctor to leave the patient. On such occasions doctors should say, "We've been keeping your mouth open for a long while. Close for a moment and rest." For those calls that can be handled, the receptionist should say, "The doctor is with a patient. May I help you?" or "May I take a number? How long will you be at that number?"

If the doctor has a lot of outside calls, a system needs to be worked out for their management. Maybe the dentist should rearrange his or her schedule so a day is available for other activities. It is harmful to the practice image and staff morale if, on a recurring basis, everything stops while the doctor chats on the telephone. Staff do not mind working late if the day has been productive. But for everyone to be late because the doctor was involved with outside activities is a sure way to produce grumbling.

Telephone disruptions are responsible for thousands of lost production dollars in dental offices. Aside from the production loss, stress is created when everyone is behind schedule. Keeping patients waiting for more than five minutes, no matter what the reason, is a detriment to practice growth. *People count up the faults of those who keep them waiting.*

Phase Two: Greeting

Every patient who enters a dental office is at least slightly apprehensive. Therefore, one of the major responsibilities of front desk personnel is to make patients feel at ease. Receptionists should be aware of the names on the appointment book, and patients should be greeted when they arrive. Patients need to relax. Small talk and compliments help. Every patient is slightly nervous, but an empathetic receptionist can resolve some of this with a reassuring manner. Make the patient feel that he or she is the most important person to walk through the office door that day. Highlight new patient names in the appointment book for easier recognition.

If staff is uncertain about the degree of formality desired in the office, the matter should be discussed with the doctor. Generally speaking, if patients are treated as if they were guests in a home, an appropriate tone is achieved. Patients are guests and deserve sincere hospitality.

As a new patient enters, the receptionist may say something like, "Good morning; you must be Mr. Black. My name is Susan. I spoke with you on the phone yesterday." This is so much nicer than, "Have a seat; I'll be with you in a moment." Introductions are great public relations tools. If the patient is new, simple manners require introducing oneself even if a nametag is being worn.

Introductions essentially say "You are important to me." There is no sweeter sound to people than the sound of their own names. Staff members should get in the habit of addressing patients by name during conversation. If the receptionist is too busy to give a warm, friendly greeting, then the office is

either understaffed or the receptionist is not the right "p
person" to have at the front desk. A warm, expressive r_eep-
tionist is vital to practice building.

When staff members greet a patient of record (remember
not to refer to established patients as "old patients"), they
should try to give a sincere compliment to that person. The
compliment must be realistic. Although compliments cheer all
patients, they are especially appreciated by children, homemakers, and the elderly. As an administrative assistant, I loved
complimenting elderly patients. We once had an elderly woman
walk in with a pretty, lavender dress (and silvered, lavender
hair to match!). In greeting this patient, I said, "Mrs. Smith, you
look lovely in that color." I do believe she walked out an inch
taller than she walked in. Compliments are good for the soul—
and for arthritic spines, as well.

Homemakers are another neglected group. Nobody pays
much attention to them unless something needs to be done.
The fact that the receptionist pays special attention could be the
highlight of the day. Small details can make big impressions.

Phase Three: Registration

Registering a patient is a simple procedure. Some offices
like to "romance" patients by filling out the forms for them. In
most offices, however, patients are asked to fill out their own
registration and health histories while waiting for their appointments. Generally, a patient would rather write the information
herself than have to verbalize such facts as that she is temporarily unemployed, that she has a bladder problem, or that she
has not seen a dentist for eight years.

Occasionally patients may forget their glasses or express the
need for assistance. Don't wait for them to call for help. The
receptionist should offer assistance by saying, "Please fill out
this information sheet, front and back, and pay particular
attention to the health questions. Dr. Wood is interested in your
total health. I'll be glad to help, if you like." Never encourage
patients to be embarrassed if they request such assistance.

The receptionist may offer coffee or juice to patients while
they are filling out the necessary forms. Many patients have
indicated via office questionnaires that this is the one "hug"
they enjoy the most about their dental office. Remember that

patients like to feel special; treat them as guests. Friendliness is essential to a good dental practice. Sometimes the only difference between one dental office and another is how the patient is welcomed and put at ease.

The first three phases of communication (telephone, greeting, and registration) take approximately ten minutes. In this short amount of time, patients have already decided if they like being part of the practice and whether they will refer their family and friends. As has been said and bears repeating, *patients only refer others to happy, attentive practices.*

Although every member of the dental team is equally important, the receptionist interacts with patients in five out of the eight patient communication phases, compared to three for the assistant or hygienist and one for the doctor. Therefore, most of the responsibility for practice-building through good communication skills rests with the receptionist.

Phase Four: Seating the Patient

This phase is normally the responsibility of the clinical staff, either the assistant or hygienist. Remember that the patient looks at the faces of the staff to determine what is going on "back there," so staff members should always wear a smile when receiving patients.

It is good for members of the clinical staff to offer introductions such as "Hello, Ms. Smith. My name is Sherry. I'm Dr. Wood's assistant." Patients want to know the staff members' names, what they do in the office, and how well they like the doctor. Although all staff should wear a name tag, the personal introduction puts the patient-assistant relationship on a friendly, caring basis. The clinical staff should not come across as plastic professionals.

In the doctor's absence, patients often ask assistants or hygienists, "Do you like working here?" or "Is he in a good mood today?" or "Why did the last assistant leave?" Patients ask such questions because their confidence in the office is related to how well the staff members and the doctor like each other. It is imperative that the staff have confidence in the doctor and in the quality of patient care being delivered in order to instill trust and reduce patients' fear.

Fear in patients is normal, and all patients need to know they are not alone in their apprehensions. After patients are seated, they should not be abandoned. If they are seated and left alone, they wonder what is going on. They do not understand being deserted. Every treatment room should have magazines suitable for men, women, and children. If it is necessary for the assistant to leave the room, the patient should be handed a magazine and an excuse made. Patients should never be left without a word of explanation. Fear and apprehension are real and tend to be magnified by the unknown.

When patients are treated as friends, they are apt to say, "That receptionist Mary at Dr. Wilson's office is *so* nice" or "Her assistant Sherry is very knowledgeable" or "Dr. Wilson's hygienist Jody really did a thorough cleaning." Such patients do not refer to staff members as the blonde, the person with the glasses, or the "cleaning lady."

Phase Five: Treatment (Doctor Time)

The doctor must always be aware of the patient's name and the reason for the visit. This information should be available on the daily work list that is present in each treatment room.

During treatment time, the chairside assistant should show concern for and interest in the patient. It is frustrating to the doctor if the assistant is preoccupied with unimportant things, looks at her watch frequently, or daydreams. Dental assisting can become repetitive, but there is a patient attached to every tooth you treat. Patients always deserve full attention nothing less.

Conversation is acceptable during treatment as long as it does not exclude or frustrate the patient because of his or her inability to join in. Small talk can be effective to relieve anxiety, but much depends on the doctor's and patient's personalities as well as the situation. The doctor and staff should never discuss personal problems in the presence of patients. Light personal conversation such as "How was your vacation?" or "I saw your daughter's wedding picture in the paper," helps build rapport. Never discuss personal problems that are "downers." In one office an assistant burdened every patient with the minute details of her divorce. Most folks have enough problems of their own. Keep conversations light.

Phase Six: Patient Education

Doctors who have trained their assistants and hygienists in patient education enjoy increased production. By turning patients over to clinical staff members, doctors ensure that rapport and confidence are built with the entire staff, not just with themselves.

The key to patient acceptance in this phase is for doctors to verbalize their trust by saying, "Ms. Johnson, it was nice seeing you. I look forward to your next visit. Sherry will be spending time with you now." The doctor can then be five to ten minutes into another procedure while being assured that Ms. Johnson is having first-class treatment from Sherry. This proper utilization of staff is not possible, however, if one dental assistant has to run back and forth between treatment rooms.

During patient education, assistants should reassure patients by telling them exactly what was done that day: "We started your root canal treatment. It is important to keep your next appointment without fail." Stressing the importance of the next appointment discourages broken appointments.

The assistant also may say, "The doctor restored seven surfaces on two teeth today. They may be sensitive to cold for several weeks. This is normal." She should never say, "If you have any *problems*, call us." Such a statement plants negative seeds and encourages problem calls. What should be said instead is "We don't expect any problems, but if you have any *questions*, feel free to call the office."

The assistant should also go over postoperative instructions and provide written instructions for extractions, periodontal surgery, and endodontic treatments. In some instances, families of patients need written information for proper home care.

Before dismissing a patient, the assistant should say, "Before you leave, Ms. Hall, are there any questions you would like to ask?" Patients often are more comfortable asking questions of staff members than of the doctor. Patients are reluctant to take the doctor's time. If the patient asks a question that the assistant does not feel comfortable in answering, she should respond, "Ms. Hall, I feel Dr. Wood should answer that question. He's with another patient at the moment. May I take a telephone number where you can be reached during the next hour? I will call you with *his* answer."

After all questions are answered, the assistant or hygienist should walk patients to within view of the desk. Then she should hand them their charts and say, "Please give your chart to Mary at the desk so she can write your receipt for today," or "so she can process your insurance form immediately." This makes collection easy: TNT (Today Not Tomorrow).

Some offices prefer that patients be escorted to the front desk. The less confusion there, the better. If the patients carry their own charts, the business staff is assured that both the charts and patients arrive back at the desk at the same time. A chronic complaint of the business staff is having patients at the desk without their charts. If this is a problem at your office, make this Golden Rule Number 1: *The dental chair cannot go into an upright position until the paperwork is completed.* Some offices have misgivings about patients carrying charts because they fear the patients will read them. Here is Golden Rule Number 2: *Never write anything in a chart you wouldn't want the patient to read.*

All instructions for posting and reappointment should be clearly written on the routing slip, computer buck-slip or quick claim by the chairside personnel. This saves times for the business staff when patients arrive at the desk. There usually are three or four clinical staff members for every business member, so the more front desk time that can be saved, the better. This may seem like a duplication of duty at chairside, but it only takes about 40 seconds of the assistant's or hygienist's time. The information is fresh on their minds after charting and saves several minutes' research per patient at the front desk.

In many offices complaints often are made about the appointment secretary and the mess the appointment book is in. Remember, however, that the routing slip or computer buck-slip is the intraoffice communicator. Therefore, the responsibility rests with the clinical staff or doctor to feed this good information to this front desk computer. As they say, "Garbage in, garbage out."

Phase Seven: Reappoint and Present Fee

At the end of each treatment, the front desk person should reappoint the patient and then present the fee for that day's treatment. By doing so, patients feel there is more concern about their continued care than their money."

In reappointing, the receptionist should ask, "Are mornings or afternoons better for you?" If the question is phrased, "When would you like to come in?" the patient might take ten minutes to decide. If the patient responds that mornings are best, the receptionist should offer a choice of two morning appointments that need to be filled by saying, "The doctor can see you Wednesday morning at 10:30 or Thursday morning at 11:00." This is how receptionists control their appointment books.

In presenting fees or setting up *payment arrangements* (do not use the term *financial arrangements,* as this smacks of retailing), the business staff should be at eye level with the patient. If the patient is standing and looking down at the business staff member, the patient has some degree of psychological control. If the business staff person has to stand to be at eye level while presenting fees, she should do so.

The business staff member will have better results when dealing with patients who have no insurance if she presents fees in positive terms such as "Your fee today is forty-five. Will that be cash, check or credit card?" If three "Yes" answers are offered, one will usually result. Never say "dollars"—it is a negative, turn-off word. The business staff member should say, "Your fee today is three twenty-five" *not* "three hundred twenty-five dollars."

Phase Eight: Exit

The last phase of patient communication, exit or dismissal, is second only to the initial telephone contact in line of importance. It is the patient's last impression of the office. The front desk person should tell the patient good-bye with words like "Ms. Jones, it was nice seeing you today. We look forward to your visit next Thursday morning at 10:00."

This phase of communication is the perfect time to double new patient referrals by inviting family, friends, and co-workers of the patient to use the practice.

If an insurance patient has good dental coverage, the receptionist may say, "Mr. Brown, I don't know if you are aware of it, but your dental plan is one of the best we see in this office. If your co-workers don't have a personal dentist, we'd be pleased to see them." Several studies have shown that 30 to 40 percent of employees with dental insurance coverage do not see dentists on a regular basis. Some of them only need to be invited.

If the office has been seeing Mrs. Johnson and her children, and she speaks of her husband, the receptionist may say, "Mrs. Johnson, we haven't had the pleasure of meeting Mr. Johnson. If he isn't seeing another dentist, we'd be glad to see him as well." It should become the goal of each staff member to invite patients to the practice. Inviting is not soliciting or recruiting; it is just being conscientious and showing concern for others.

Positive Words Equal Positive Results

At several points in this book, I have identified words and phrases we should or should not use in the dental setting. Communicating in a positive manner with patients and one another is of utmost importance to the growth of the practice.

One of my pet peeves is the use of negative words in dental offices. From the negative signs in the reception area that turn off the patients to the negative retail words used in presenting fees, the words we use have a powerful effect on the patients' emotions.

Table 4–1 lists "Do Say and Don't Say" phrases to enhance the odds for patients having positive experiences at the dental office. This list should be studied often because old habits can be difficult to change.

Words that should never be said include "expensive" and "whoops!" Doctors should never be addressed by their first names in front of patients.

Handling Difficult Patients

The adage that "2 percent of the patients cause 98 percent of the stress" is frequently true. Don't dwell on the 2 percent. Rather, tune in on the 98 percent, the wonderful patients, and learn to deal with the two-percenters.

If a patient sits in the chair and complains about his or her past dentists, there is little doubt that the present dentist will be the next one on that person's long list. Be a good listener, but beware.

Table 4–1 Do Say and Don't Say Phrases

Do Say	Don't Say	Why
Reception Room	Waiting Room	Implies we keep our patients waiting
Treatment room	Operatory	Sounds like we are going to operate
Consultation room	Private office	No one is allowed
Necessary X-rays	Full mouth series	Makes gaggers want to gag
May I tell the doctor who is calling?	May I ask who is calling?	Sounds nosey
Treatment or dentistry	Work	Could mean anything
Sedative or medicated restoration	Temporary filling	Shouldn't be a fee if replaced
Follow-up care or preventive program	Checkup or recall	Sounds insignificant (cars are recalled)
Prepare or reshape the tooth	Grind the tooth	Scares the patients
Primary teeth	Baby teeth	Immature speech
The assistant or staff	The girls	Sounds derogatory
Fee	Price or charge	Retail words
Statement	Bill	Less professional
Payment arrangements	Financial arrangements	Too retail
Take care of	Pay for	Too retail
Agreement	Contract or note	Too rigid
Investment	Cost	Sounds retail
Your fee today is forty-five	Your fee today is forty-five *dollars*	"Dollars" is negative

Table 4–1 (Cont.)

Do Say	Don't Say	Why
Your crown is three-fifty	Your Crown is three *hundred* fifty *dollars*	"Hundreds" and "dollars" sound higher
Bookkeeper's allowance or professional courtesy or senior citizen courtesy	Discount	Cheapens your practice; sounds like a discount store
Patient of record	Old patient	Few people want to be an "old" anything
Thorough examination	Checkup	Air of competency
Uncomplicated extraction	Simple extraction	Should not have much of a fee if simple
Do you prefer mornings or afternoons?	When would you like to come in?	May take ten minutes for them to decide
Doctor has had an interruption in his schedule	Doctor is running late	Sounds as if he is out jogging
We're looking forward to seeing you tomorrow at 11:00	I'm calling to remind you of your appointment tomorrow at 11:00	Makes patients feel feeble-minded
Change in schedule	Cancellation	Creates holes in the schedule (okay to cancel)
How do you feel about this?	Do you understand?	Makes patients feel dumb
Call by number	Chisel or forceps	Frightens patients
Call by color	Syringe needle	Frightens patients
Discomfort	Hurt or pain	Conjures pain

beware.

Many two-percenters do not intend to be stress-creators; they just are. The following are examples of nonintentional stress-creators.

The Frightened Patient

When these patients call the office, they may say to the receptionist, "I hate going to the dentist; it has taken me three years to make this call" or "I'm scared to death of dentists; my last experience was terrible." Such expressions of high fear–low trust should be noted and believed—fear is real!

When you are making appointments, if patients admit that it is difficult for them to come to the dentist, mark their names in the appointment book in such a manner that all the staff will know they need some extra time and attention. Mark "TLC" by the name for "Tender, Loving Care" and everyone will know the patient needs to feel especially welcome and reassured. Kindness and concern go farther with a patient than comments such as "You have nothing to worry about—you will be fine." Neither the patient nor the staff really know that everything will be fine until the treatment is done. Don't make empty promises; they undermine the patient's trust.

In alleviating the patient's apprehension chairside, don't say, "Oh, Mr. Jones, there's nothing to a root canal—in fact, it's no worse than a filling." This, in fact, creates higher fear and lower trust and makes the patient feel he is being treated like a child.

Any time a patient expresses feelings of fear, it should be noted on the chart. Some offices identify this with red medic alert tape on the outside of their charts and a notation of TLC. It means this patient is always nervous and needs more than the usual amount of tender, loving care.

In my appointment book I noted "NP (TLC)," which meant the new patient expressed high fear and low trust and needs extra TLC. I feel everyone in the office needs to be aware of this potential problem patient. If the notation is written on the appointment book before the patient comes in, the front desk person can place it on the worklist the day before and thereby alert the entire staff to the NP (TLC). If the office has staff meetings at the beginning of the day's schedule, such patients can be identified at that time.

New staff members need to be instructed to never try to talk frightened patients out of fear—it only heightens it. Instead, staff members should be sympathetic to feelings by saying, "We have a word that describes how you feel, Mr. Jones. That word is *normal.*" Patients begin to relax when they feel they arc understood; they feel safer and more secure.

The Late Patient

Patients cannot be expected to be on time if they have been kept waiting to see the dentist in the past. I find in office after office that prompt patients acquire their good habits from offices that truly respect their time. On the other hand, in offices that consistently run behind schedule, late patients and cancellations are prevalent.

Chronic tardiness is nothing but a bad habit. Unforeseen events and emergencies can disrupt the schedule of any dental office once in a while. But if such things happen more than 10 percent of the time, causes need to be determined and actions taken to correct the problem. Patients get their habits from office practices. Let us examine tardiness in several instances.

Show me doctors who are late for work every day or late coming back from lunch, and I will show you doctors who would rather be somewhere else. Their heart is not in dentistry. This behavior demonstrates both to staff and patients that there is a motivational problem at the top. How can the staff be motivated to be on time and feel good about their jobs when doctors don't feel good about theirs?

Cavett Robert, founder of the National Speaker's Association, says, "Success is finding something you enjoy doing so much you would do it for free, but doing it so well you get paid for it." Being late every day is not a sign of satisfaction and success.

In one office I visited, a doctor would not allow patients to be seated until they had waited for *him* at least ten minutes— even if he was only reading the paper while they waited. My observation of that situation was that a big ego problem existed. Such a policy is indicative of either a tragic insecurity or an enormous misappraisal of one's own importance.

It is embarrassing for the staff to be compelled to continually make excuses for their doctor's tardiness. It is also a big production killer.

In another office the doctor had a problem of visiting for about 15 minutes with each of his two hygienists' patients. This wonderful doctor loves his work and his patients, but he simply loses track of time. As a matter of fact, when questioned about this habit, he thought he spent about three minutes with each patient. His schedule was booked solid for weeks because he kept postponing half of what he had been planning as a result of visiting too long with the hygienists' patients.

Because he lost track of time entirely, I told his staff to buy two huge three-minute egg timers. When the dentist walks into the hygiene room, the hygienist quietly turns the egg timer behind the patient. When the sand is in the bottom, the doctor knows his hygiene check should be over.

With competent hygienists on staff, dentists should not have to spend fifteen minutes checking patients. There will be instances, of course, where this more efficient routine cannot be followed. But interestingly enough, with improved time habits this particular office's productivity increased hundreds of dollars per day. I am not saying a dentist should not visit and chat with patients. But trained staff can share in this important phase of patient care and in the process save the doctor's productive time. At $200 to $250 per hour, saving ten minutes per patient per day in a practice that sees twenty patients will increase daily income by $600 to $800.

Any dental office that expects its patients to be on time for their appointments must have policies that demonstrate to the patient that their time is also respected and considered valuable. The following policies have proven effective in this regard.

Policy 1. If the doctor or hygienist is five minutes late, the receptionist is responsible for acknowledging such tardiness to the patient with an apology. Only waiting patients who are ignored are hostile. I have found that patients to whom apologies are made are understanding and tolerant of short waits.

Policy 2. If the doctor or hygienist is ten minutes late, he or she must go into the reception room and apologize *in person* to the waiting patient. With these policies in force, I can guarantee that the office will never be more than 9½ minutes late.

There will always be some tardy patients regardless of the policies of the practice. Here are a few tips that help:

1. If a patient is habitually late, I recommend writing the time of the appointment 15 minutes earlier on the appointment card than in the appointment book, for example, 10:45 on the card and 11:00 in the book. A question arises: "What if, for instance, they are on time for once?" Answer: "They have kept the office waiting so many times in the past, it is okay to make them wait until they develop better time habits."

2. Have the following message printed on the patient brochure and appointment cards: "We try to see our patients on time and appreciate the same promptness from our patients."

3. Develop an office policy that doctors and staff are comfortable with for managing very tardy patients. I recommend rescheduling patients if they are late for more than half their appointment times. For instance, if a patient has a 40-minute appointment in the hygiene department and shows up 25 minutes late, the patient probably should be rescheduled. In such instances the hygienist has three options: (1) elect to do half the prophy and reschedule the rest, (2) do a rush job in half the allotted time, or (3) reschedule the patient for another time. Rescheduling is usually the best choice.

   Attempts to see patients are apt to be stressful. Patients who receive half a prophy may be angered by such treatment. Patients who get very fast treatment may say to the dentist, "Well, I certainly hope I don't get such a rush job on my next appointment." Rescheduling is usually best. If patients are alienated by the truth, they probably were not very friendly to begin with.

There are two ways to manage a dental office: with policies or without. If there are no policies—if the patients decide when and if they are coming and when and if they will pay—chaos and stress prevail. In order to have a happy environment that the dentist, staff, and patients look forward to, I highly recommend setting policies and guidelines. Paul Jacobi, in his

Flight Manual to Success, states, "An airline shouldn't fly without a flight plan and neither should your dental office." Policies are flight plans.

Chapter **5**

Time Management

Being organized with a simple time management system can add much satisfaction to one's life. The joy of feeling a true sense of accomplishment leads to a happier, more productive dental office.

This chapter addresses the time-wasters in one's business and personal life and offers solutions for dealing with interruptions on a day-to-day basis.

In the dental office, good time management systems are essential if the office is to be productive. The profit margin of the practice is directly proportionate to the way the dental team manages its time.

Time Management/Self-Management

We have 24 hours to spend each day. Many people think they should try to save time. That is impossible. You can't buy it, change it, save it, or borrow it. Time can only be spent. The question, really, is *how* it is going to be spent. With simple time management tips, you can start spending time more productively. By doing so, more time becomes available for things that we keep putting off. Time management ideas seem to make more hours available every day. Time passes despite our pleas or prayers, but time management techniques allow some control over the process.

I use a three-item list. Since adopting this system, I find I accomplish much more with my time. Don't think you are too busy to develop a three-item list system. The old adage "If you want something done, go to a busy person" is true. Busy people are productive people *because* they are organized.

At the end of each day, I make my three-item list for the next day. This takes about five minutes daily but conserves many hours each week. The lists include the following:

1. **To Do List.** The things I want to do tomorrow. Those that are most urgent should be listed first and numbered in order of priority of importance.
2. **To Call List.** The people I must call tommorrow to make things happen, or whose calls must be returned.
3. **To Go List.** The errands I must run such as to the bank, insurance company, or lawyer's office.

Mark off the items on the list as they are finished. This brings feelings of accomplishment and satisfaction, besides allowing more work to be completed each day.

Learn to set priorities for your work. Priority is not necessarily what is on the top of the stack, but rather those tasks which have deadlines. There is a temptation to do the fun and easy things first, leaving the more difficult work until last. Such work patterns only expand frustration.

Procrastination creates stress. When you have a big job, remember that "You can only eat an elephant one bite at a time." Start nibbling at a job and watch it disappear.

Writing this book was a big task that I kept placing on the back burner. By using the excuse that I was too busy, I was able to put it off for a long time. I assured both myself and others that this excuse was legitimate and beyond my ability to change. It wasn't until my editor read my first chapters and said "You have a message—get with it; your deadline is in four months" that I decided to tackle the project seriously.

With a completely filled consulting and speaking schedule and a family, how was I going to find the time to write a book by the deadline? I took the advice of my mentor, Mary Kay Ashe, founder of Mary Kay Cosmetics. According to her, successful people always find the time to do important things.

She talks about the "five o'clock club." I have never been an early riser. To get up at 5:00 A.M., especially in winter months, was a real chore at first. After a while, I actually learned to like it. Now my routine is to write from 5:00 to 6:30 A.M., jog or walk for 30 minutes, shower, and then get to work by 8:30. It has been wonderful! I plan to write a second book soon.

You, too, can accomplish more than you ever imagined if you write it down and then go for it. The old saying "plan your work, and then work your plan" is the secret of time management.

Make weekly plans on Friday for the coming week. Again, I recommend the three-item list, but for the entire week. This plan takes about ten minutes on Friday but will greatly increase your effectiveness and ability to get things done.

Reward yourself when you meet your objectives and deadlines on important projects. The reward should fit the task. For example, suppose you love pizza but know it is laden with unwanted calories. At the end of the month, if you finish each week's list of "to do," "to call," and "to go," reward yourself with your favorite pizza. You can go back on your diet the next day.

Avoid interruptions. It has been estimated that the average person is interrupted 40 to 60 times per day. In a dental office, the front desk staff learns to work with interruptions. They are interrupted 100 to 150 times a day with telephone calls, patients coming and going, and the needs of the doctor and the rest of the staff. This is why I advocate written communications from the back office to the front desk. It reduces front desk interruptions by as much as 40 to 50%.

The telephone is the biggest source of interruption in business. To save time with telephoning, make a note of the things you need to discuss, avoid trivial comments, and end the call when the conversation is over. Tell long-winded callers you have another call waiting (some people don't know how to say good-bye). When placing a call or answering one, start the conversation with, "Oh, Mary, I'm glad you caught me—I was just on my way to an important meeting" or "While my patient is getting numb, I want to spend a couple of minutes discussing Ms. Jones's periodontal progress." If doctors and staff totaled the number of wasted production hours caused by improper use of the telephone, they would be astounded by the number of dollars lost.

Firm policies regarding personal telephone calls have added as much as $200 per day to the production of dental offices— more than $40,000 per year. If the office has a policy of no incoming personal calls except for family emergencies, then staff and doctors must abide by the policy. If 7 people in an office have 3 personal calls each, it amounts to 21 interruptions per day for the receptionist. Family and friends should be instructed not to call during patient hours. It also is unfair to the patients who are trying to reach the office. Doctors should not ask staff members to adopt good time management habits until they, the leaders, do so.

At the next staff meeting, have each person write her or his name and title on the top of a sheet of paper. Then pose the question, "What does this person do that wastes my time?" Pass each paper around to all staff members for their comments. Each person writes down what the other team members do that wastes their time. This exercise is a real eye-opener in most offices. These time-wasters should be read aloud and discussed by the staff. Gentle criticism boosts production and helps us build a better, more effective team.

Delegating to Others

Dentists who know how to delegate enjoy the highest productivity levels and the least amount of stress. Office administrators can relieve doctors of many management details. If state law allows a duty to be delegated to someone of a lesser salary, it should be. State dental practice acts should be reviewed to determine the maximum allowable use of expanded duty auxiliaries. Successful delegating includes the following:

1. Clear and specific instructions. Staff members should not be expected to guess or to read minds. Written guidelines save time and stress.
2. Encouragement to use personal knowledge and skills. When I hire a new staff member, I go over the history of our firm, its philosophy, and its long- and short-term goals. Then I say, "Tomorrow bring a list of three ways you feel you can help us meet these goals by using your

personal knowledge and skills." There is much hidden talent in employees that goes untapped for lack of inquiry.

Not long ago I hired a secretary to help with inquiries and shipping labels. I subsequently learned she had tremendous research and organizational skills. I delegated the shipping duties to a part-time secretary and channeled the person originally hired for these tasks into marketing and public relations. Big dividends resulted for all.

People do much better jobs if they like what they are doing. I hire only sharp people who know their jobs better than I do. There are unused abilities on the staff of every practice. It is in everyone's interest for these abilities to come to the surface. Someone on staff may be great at writing a quarterly newsletter, another may excel at purging inactive patient files, and someone else may be super at organizing the inventory or collecting past-due accounts.

3. Expressions of confidence and appreciation. Staff members should be complimented for accepting delegated tasks and praised when they perform well.
4. The avoidance of dictatorial directives. Participative management motivates staff to excellence and peak performance. Delegation that fails to allow individual input has the opposite effect.
5. Provision of adequate authority to fulfill the task. Many offices discuss good ideas after a seminar or consultation but never implement them because the boss won't release enough authority for their fulfillment.

Those in positions of authority must determine the manner in which they will manage the efforts of others. Management styles include the following:

1. Look at the problem; report all the facts to me. I will decide what to do.
2. Look at the problem, get all the facts, and recommend a solution. I will decide whether it is good.

3. Look at the problem; let me know what you intend to do. Let's discuss it before you take action.
4. Take action; let me know how you handled it.
5. Take action. No further contact with me is necessary.

If a staff member comes aboard who has always operated on Level 4 or 5 and the doctor is most comfortable with Level 1 or 2, the prospects for a successful working relationship are not very good. The staff member will not feel trusted. The doctor should hire someone who is at ease accepting responsibility.

If a passive person is hired for a position of responsibility and authority, the prospects for a management problem are high. In this situation the employee is always waiting for directions before proceeding with his or her task. When hiring employees, you should try to determine the applicants' assertiveness levels. This can help prevent a mismatched working relationship.

Paperwork Tips

Eliminating wasted time by proper handling of paperwork is essential to good time management. Paperwork consumes many hours of time in every office. With some effort and organization, it can be streamlined.

Mail Handling
There are three types of mail:

1. That which requires action sooner or later.
2. Journals, magazines, and newsletters to be read later.
3. Junk mail to be thrown away now.

Letter Writing
A good policy with letters is "in today and out tomorrow." There are three ways to handle letters that need a response.

1. Dictate a response at the time the letter is read.
2. Jot a short note at the bottom of the letter for a secretary to develop into a response.
3. Use a form letter from the word processors when possible.

General Files

In most dental offices, tons of paper accumulate over years of practice. Many times little, if any, of that material is ever used.

Certified public accountants and legal advisors can tell you how long tax and business files must be retained. The state insurance commissioner's office can advise how long insurance files should be kept. The state employment commission can provide a list of what records must be retained for past employees, present staff, and job applicants. A little time spent securing this information and incorporating it in the policy manual could save hours and stress in the event of an audit or other need to produce records.

General files of a business nature should be packed away at the end of the calendar year. Such records should be kept in file boxes with the year and contents clearly marked on the end of each box. Have a house-cleaning party every year after New Year's. At our office, it is called a G.I. party—gee, I wish I were doing something else! Getting the general files prepared for the coming year is a large but necessary task.

With magazines and journals, I recommend that doctors highlight their favorite articles in the table of contents and then have a staff member clip and file them in appropriately labeled folders such as TMJ, bonding, or insurance. An enormous amount of space is required to keep old journals. It is usually an unrealistic decision.

Many people would be embarrassed if others saw how their desks look most of the time. As they say, "A clean desk is a sign of a clean mind, and a cluttered desk is the sign of a busy mind." But the fact remains that anyone can be more productive in an organized work area. I recommend this: go to your office on a Saturday or Sunday when no one else is there. Dump the contents of all the drawers on top of the desk. Have a large wastebasket for things that need to be discarded. Put everything else away in a very neat fashion. Most people report having found things that had been lost for some time when they follow this suggestion.

Personal Time Management

If more personal time were available, how would you spend it? Some people would just watch more TV. I once heard that the fewer hours a person watches TV, the more successful they become. It has been said that "the way we spend our time determines how we live our lives." That's a thought.

I recommend keeping a personal time log for one week. Make a record of the amount of time spent eating, working, with spouse and family, sleeping, socializing, worshipping, and in self-improvement activities such as studying, reading, listening to tapes, or exercising.

Then determine what percent of your time is spent in each category. To get the percentages, add all the hours for the week in each category, divide by 7, and then divide again by 24.

> **Example:**
>   2.5 hours/day eating × 7 = 17.5 for the week
>   17.5 ÷ 7 days/week ÷ 24 hours/day = 10.4
>   percent of your time spent eating
>   7.5 hours/day sleeping × 7 = 52.5 hours for
>   the week
>   52.5 ÷ 7 days/week ÷ 24 hours/day = 31.2
>   percent of your time spent sleeping

Ask yourself this question: Did you enjoy the time you spent in each category? If you did not, try to figure out how to eliminate the things you dislike in order to make room for those you do.

While attending the Pankey Institute in Miami, I had the opportunity to hear Dr. L.D. Pankey speak about the need to achieve balance in our lives. According to Dr. Pankey, we should spend 25 percent of our time working, 25 percent in rest and spiritual activities, 25 percent with family and loved ones, and 25 percent in play or self-improvement. I realized that, by these criteria, my life at that time was out of balance. Back then my work was consuming approximately 60 percent of my time. Realizing this was jeopardizing my family, health, and well-being, I worked to get my life back in better balance.

If you love your work as I do, it becomes almost a hobby. But workaholics steal from personal relationships and responsibilities. Rejoice if you love your work, but learn to delegate and to recognize the importance of achieving balance in how you spend your time. I am satisfied that I am now more productive, healthier, and happier than when my life was out of balance.

Sit down today and list your goals. Doctors and staff should all list the following one- and five-year goals. Goals go into motion after you write them down and share them with at least three other people. Here are the goals to write about:

1. Career
2. Family
3. Personal development
4. Financial
5. Spiritual
6. Leisure

On your birthday, pull out the goal sheet for reevaluation. If you are married, have your spouse do the same exercise. It can add zest to your marriage and give your relationship new meaning.

Develop a time management plan today. Remember, time can't be saved—only spent. Stop worrying about trying to save time and start thinkng about how to spend it more wisely.

Scheduling

Proper patient scheduling is a problem that confronts every dental practice. Keeping all members of the dental office working as a team can be a juggling act. Following are some of the factors that handicap proper scheduling.

Understaffing

A good rule of thumb for proper clinical staffing is to have a clinical staff person for each dental chair. Many offices lose hundreds of dollars daily as a result of understaffing or improperly utilizing the staff they have. In many offices, one dental assistant is required to take care of two rooms of patients. Such staffing policies are rarely effective.

Other offices wonder why they can't keep a front desk person for very long, never realizing that one staff member is being asked to do the work of two people. Useful guidelines for determining the number of staff needed are (1) a clinical person for each dental chair and (2) a business person for every $20,000 of monthly production.

Underequipping

Underequipping can be a serious disadvantage. It occurs in several forms.

Old, outdated equipment has no place in a modern dental office. Such equipment not only slows down the operators but causes the patients to wonder if the office is behind in the latest dental techniques. Purchasing used equipment as a temporary measure can be justified if it is in good repair, functions properly, and is replaced as soon as production allows. It is false economy to skimp on equipment because it will only result in lost production.

An inadequate number of instruments is another handicap in clinical efficiency. All treatment rooms should be adequately equipped with similar setups. There should be no favorites when it comes to working areas. With all the current health risks facing dental patients and the dental team, there is more need than ever to ensure that the treatment rooms are adequately equipped with properly sterilized instruments.

Underutilizing Staff

Delegating all duties allowed by state law and proper scheduling can make a significant difference in daily production levels. Why should there be two dental assistants if one is waiting for the doctor 40 to 50 percent of the time? All staff members should remember two phrases:

1. Every time you see an empty dental chair, consider yourself temporarily unemployed.
2. When the patient's mouth closes, production stops.

Many dentists have never learned how to delegate. As a consequence, talented staff members sometimes get bored and look for other jobs, frequently outside dentistry. As leaders, dentists must hire, train, and then trust. Trust is often the link that is missing in the dental work triangle.

Before doctors can delegate, they must fix the word "trust" in their minds. When doctors accept and trust their staff, so will the patients. I have heard dentists say, "I don't have a hygienist because my patients don't like hygienists." I always smile to myself and think, "Guess who else doesn't like hygienists?"

Slow-Moving Doctors and Staff

Some doctors and staff are turtles when it comes to the way they function. I have met dentists who like to anesthetize a patient, then go read the newpaper, have a cup of coffee, and smoke a cigarette A lot of these dentists then complain because their production is low.

A great deal of stress results when a tortoise dentist hires a hare staff—one that likes to move quickly, provide excellent care, and get out on time for lunch and at the end of the day. Equally frustrating is when a hare or goal-oriented doctor accidentally hires one or more slow-moving staff members. Careful employment interviewing will minimize these incompatibilities.

Small Thinkers

Beware of dental team players who think small. Their built-in calculators (brain) may never go beyond a $20,000 monthly production figure. For such persons, "good enough" is the byword and "goals" is a term used by crazy people.

I am always amazed by how often practices double their production when they double their goals. Losers always blame circumstances for their poor results. "We always have a bad December. People are saving their money for the holidays, you know" or "The practice will never do more than $15,000 a month—we're rural." In the first instance, December should be a banner month because of patients taking advantage of their current year's insurance coverages. And some of the most successful practices I know are rural. We become what we think we are.

I tell the doctors and staff I meet, "You can become anything you want—if you believe it." The old adage that "The body achieves what the mind believes" is true. My advice to small thinkers is to visit successful practices. Become involved at different social levels. If all the friends you associate with have loser's excuses, you will too until you remove yourself from that level of thinking. Sound impossible? Try it and see.

Appointment Book Control

A major handicap to correct scheduling is not having the right kind of appointment book. The appointment book should have a column for each chair. Schedule patients in each column in an organized fashion. Doctor time must be scheduled opposite auxiliary time. My personal preference is an appointment book that is divided into ten-minute intervals.

In training new appointment receptionists to double-book the doctor's two chairs, I recommend placing all primary treatment procedures (those which require the attendance of the doctor) in Column 1 and all secondary treatment procedures (those that can be legally delegated to an auxiliary) in Column 2. Restorative procedures can be scheduled in Column 2, but only during those time intervals when the first chairside assistant is performing delegated procedures in Column 1.

There are many manual systems for designating doctor time and auxiliary time. The easiest system is to have the doctor mark a red pencil line in Column 1 showing the new receptionist where the doctor is during treatment.

"Filler appointments" are treatments that can be delegated to the second chairside assistant. Before delegating, however, be certain state laws allow for the performance of the procedure in question. New patient interviews by the second dental assistant in the time slot opposite the doctor's busy time in Chair 1 can boost production hundreds of dollars per day. Other filler appointments that can be scheduled in Chair 2 are "look-sees," postoperatives, suture removals, denture adjustments, full-mouth X-rays, and the placements of temporaries.

It is easier to handle an appointment book if it is positioned on a 45-degree ledge on the desk. This angles the book in such a way as to reduce the glare from overhead lights. In addition, the position leaves space for the pegboard beneath it.

Dental assistants are allowed to interview patients in most states. Therefore, they should assist the doctor on the patient's first visit. We have found that patients accept staff only if doctors show they trust the staff. If Mary just walks in and begins a preliminary interview and examination, the patient may wonder who she is. A simple introduction—by the doctor—sets the stage for patient acceptance of the team approach. The patient then can be rescheduled for a prophy after the appropriate amount of time has been determined.

The following is an example of a new-patient interview performed by a trained chairside assistant. This can turn the second chair into a highly productive area while the doctor and hygienist are treating patients in other rooms.

The doctor should walk into the treatment room with the second assistant, introduce himself or herself, and then say, "This is Sherry, my assistant, whom you've already met. I have asked her to spend some time with you now. She will be asking some very important questions, taking the necessary X-rays, and getting other pertinent data. As soon as she is finished, I'll be back for a thorough examination." The doctor then returns to work in another treatment room.

Sherry, with a very caring manner, sits in the doctor's chair with the chart on her lap. The attitude of the interviewer is very important. He or she can make new patients feel as if they are the only ones being treated that day. Best of all, this frees the doctor hundreds of hours per month.

Sherry begins the interview with two very important questions, noting the patient's answers on the chart. The first one is "Mr. Stephens, before we do anything else, tell me how you feel about your teeth." We can talk to patients endlessly about what they *need*, but people only buy what they *want*.

Mr. Stephens may say, "Well, my parents both lost their teeth around age 35. I am now 33. I guess it's about time for me to lose mine." Or he may say "My parents both lost their teeth at an early age, and I will do everything I can to keep mine."

The second question that should be asked is, "Is there anything about your smile you don't like?" Many people don't like their smiles and would like to change them. Cosmetic dentistry alone could keep most dental offices busy if only it were recommended to patients. That is why the staff should be trained to assist with the new patient interview.

If patients first hear their dental needs identified by the dentist, they think "money." But if staff members have asked positive questions that led into a dental discussion and the doctor then reinforced the need, the patients think "concern." A point to keep in mind when interviewing new patients is that staff members can never diagnose; only doctors can. But staff members can ask questions that plant positive seeds of need.

After reviewing the health questions with the patient, Sherry marks in red pencil any medical problems that have been identified. She places red medic alert tape on the outside of the patient's chart for instant referral to the medical problem. She then does the blood pressure screening and charts the existing restorations.

Of course, charting existing restorations isn't absolutely necessary, but it gives staff members an opportunity to view the patient's dental condition. It does not require the highly skilled talents of a dentist or hygienist to spot obvious problems such as missing teeth, fractured or missing restorations, poor hygiene, or rampant decay. In charting existing restorations in gray lead pencil, the assistant should ask questions such as "Has anyone ever mentioned replacing this lower first molar, Mr. Stephens?" or "Does the edge of this fractured tooth bother you?"

After the assistant charts the existing restorations, she can have before-and-after visual aids in the treatment room to show the patient while she develops the X-rays. Dr. Ross Nash's *Cosmetic Dentistry Photo Book* (actual before-and-after photographs), or Dr. Ronald Goldstein's book *Change Your Smile* are excellent patient motivators. Every time X-rays are processed in the office, before-and-after photos of the particular patient's needs should be made available to the patient.

When the doctor walks into the treatment room for the complete examination, time is saved if everything is organized and ready. The chart should be placed beside the sink. As the doctor washes his or her hands, the chart can be read. The patient's likes and dislikes, feelings about his or her teeth, blood pressure, medical information, and charting, can be presented to the doctor.

The doctor should do a soft tissue examination, oral cancer examination, occlusal evaluations, and periodontal probing. Using simple terminology, the doctor calls off exactly what Mr. Stephens needs on teeth 1 through 32. Recommended nondental terms include "chewing surface," "cheek side," "tongue side," "front" and "back."

After the doctor has called off teeth 1 through 32, Sherry reads back the information to ensure it is charted correctly. This also serves as double reinforcement for the patient. On smaller treatment plans, the case discussion should be held chairside rather than with a full consultation. On larger cases, the full consultation is a necessity.

Many staff members say, "This new-patient interview *must* be done by a hygienist because our patients want their teeth cleaned on the first appointment." This is a good point, but how does the receptionist know how much time to schedule for the cleaning? I recommend that on the first telephone contact the receptionist say, "Our new patient examination consists of _____, _____, and _____. You will be rescheduled in our hygiene department after the doctor's examination has determined the amount of time you need."

On rare occasions a patient will say, "I'm in a wedding in ten days and I thought I should get my teeth cleaned." Try to accommodate that patient by dovetailing the appointments: 30 minutes with the second dental assistant and 30 minutes with the hygienist. If dovetailing is not possible, the hygienist may see the new patient.

This type of triple booking allows more new patients to be seen immediately. People who call the office as nonemergency new patients should be seen within three or four days. Because this saves time for the hygienist, it allows more time for recalls and initial periodontal treatments.

Reports indicate that more than 75 percent of dental patients have beginning to advanced periodontal disease. A talented hygienist should spend the day treating and reeducating patients in the hygiene department. One of the few ways to increase production in dentistry is to delegate to someone at a lesser salary those duties that can be legally performed by auxiliary personnel.

Another system of improving productivity is to have two hygiene chairs and a hygienist-assistant team. Patient's appointments are staggered, allowing the hygienist to do the scaling, patient education, and selling. The assistant does the seating, X-rays, polishing (in some states), home care instruction, and reappointing. This "dynamic duo" system is quite effective if you have the space (chairs), patient load, and a team dedicated to results and volume.

It surprises me to find dentists still doing prophys. They say, "If I don't do prophys about 50 hours a month, I won't be busy." This statement has been proven wrong time and again.

When the hygienist sees all the prophys and sets the stage for case acceptance, the doctor's 50 hours are spent doing restorative work instead of duties that can be delegated. I have seen dozens of offices double their production when proper delegation was practiced.

Many dentists hire staff but do not fully train or trust them to do this preliminary new-patient interview. I have seen staff members blossom when they were trusted with more responsibility in patient communication. The production increases from the first day. It is not always easy, but keep in mind that a new system only works when everyone in the office says, "Let's make it work!"

Increases in production are the result of the entire team working together, dividing the responsibilities, and selling quality dentistry. If people on the staff are concentrating on their own plans or problems instead of on the patient's needs, the continuity of the office's attitude is interrupted. One hitch in the patient flow disrupts the pace and can send a signal to the patient that he or she is not the most important person in the office. When the duties and responsibilities are equitably divided among the staff members, everyone feels that his or her contribution to the practice is essential. More business walks out of some offices than other offices see in their lifetime.

Reducing No-Shows and Broken Appointments

Reducing no-shows and broken appointments is a matter of attitude and communication. In offices that have no built-in extra time for busy work—what I call "tooth fairy time"—staff members not only accept a patient's excuses for changing and breaking appointments but, in some cases, subconsciously encourage them. As a former staff member, I can understand and appreciate these nonintentional negative attitudes. If there is never any time to do the busy work, and stacks begin to grow stacks, it is not difficult to learn to like no-shows and last-minute broken appointments.

I have observed, however, that offices that do adopt "tooth fairy time" have fewer holes in their schedules. That is because their staff feel free to devote their full attention to treating patients.

At the monthly staff meeting, the front desk person's report should include the number of patients who tried to change or break appointments as well as the number who were convinced to keep their appointments. This record is kept at the bottom of the appointment book each day by making an X for each attempted change or cancellation. If the appointment is maintained that day, circle the X.

An average dental practice can be 15 to 30 percent more productive if it eliminates the holes in doctors' and hygienists' schedules. When a good receptionist receives a call changing the schedule, she walks to the treatment room, lines through a name, writes CA for canceled appointment, and then places another name above the one lined through. In other words, the doctor's or hygienist's problem is solved before he or she even knew there was one.

A sign of a not-so-efficient receptionist is someone who walks to the work lists, lines through two or more names, writes CA, and announces, "Well, we had a good day planned, but we just had three changed appointments. It looks like we have no patients from 10:30 to 2:00. Enjoy your long lunch." This person then returns to the business area to work on piled-up insurance forms, which should not be top priority or, for that matter, even accumulated.

Like any skill, the art of discouraging broken appointments or last-minute changes can be developed. You first must learn to distinguish between the worthwhile reasons for changes and those which are but feeble excuses. Most patients with worthwhile reasons call very early in the morning. Such patients begin the conversation with an apology: "Gee, I'm so sorry I must change my appointment today, but my baby was up all night with an earache and her doctor's appointment is the same time as my dental appointment."

In handling this situation, the receptionist should say, "I know how that is, Mrs. White. I understand completely. Rather than take up your time now, I'll make a note to call you before 5:00 this afternoon to reschedule your appointment and to inquire about the baby." This demonstrates true concern, not only for the patient but for her child as well.

On the other hand, you'll want to change your strategy if a patient calls with a feeble excuse such as, "I didn't know it would be a sunny day, and I've decided to go to the beach," or

"The soap opera is getting good; I'd like to change my appointment to a morning time" or "I have a problem with my car."

If a patient puts hair appointments, beach weather, and soap operas on a higher priority list than a dental appointment, make rescheduling difficult. Never give a feeble-excuse patient the next available time, or "prime time" privileges. In these cases an appropriate response is, "The doctor can see you in eight to ten weeks." The primary cause of broken appointments is that in too many offices they are accepted as part of the normal day.

The first step in eliminating most of the holes in your schedule is to discourage wasted time. The best defense is a good offense. If the staff learns a few tactics, many of the holes can be filled. Following are a few effective techniques:

1. When patients try to cancel or postpone their appointments, sound disappointed yet nice. It is possible to be friendly and disappointed at the same time.

2. When scheduling a patient for the next appointment, stress the importance of that visit, such as, "Your root canal treatment was started today. For best results, it is very important to keep your next appointment as scheduled." Or "You should have no problems with your temporary crown. However, it is important that you return in three weeks as scheduled." Many patients feel they can postpone treatment if they are not having a problem.

3. Make rescheduling difficult for those with feeble excuses, as when a mother says, "Little Jimmy has soccer practice, so I'd like to change all four of my children's appointments." At such a moment, you should create a new office policy by saying, "Gee, Ms. Brown, I'm so sorry you can't keep these appointments since we usually, just for this reason, don't grant multiple family appointments. In the future, I'm sure you'll understand why we can no longer see your family at one time and will have to schedule their appointments one at a time." Little Jimmy will miss soccer practice, or three out of the four appointments will be kept.

For other poor excuses say, "I'm sorry you can't keep that appointment tomorrow with Susan, our hygienist. Her next available time is in three months."

The usual response is, "Oh, in that case, I'd better keep it." I found that when I showed disappointment and made rescheduling difficult, I could talk more than 60 percent of the feeble-excuse patients into keeping their appointments. Patients like being accommodated for their own convenience, so this policy works wonders for irresponsible patients.

4. Find a solution to the patient's problem in a very courteous manner. For example, if a patient had a two-hour crown and bridge appointment and attempted to cancel or postpone due to a car problem (always a good excuse, in the patient's opinion), say, "To preserve this valuable time on the doctor's schedule, the office will be glad to send a cab."

I must have offered 30 taxies during my last year at the desk, but no one ever took me up on it. They always said, "Oh, I bet my neighbor, or the secretary at the next desk, will give me a ride." People only keep appointments they want to keep. The challenge is to make the patients want to please you. Showing disappointment in a friendly manner is the key to reducing wasted hours each day. The receptionist's tone of voice either encourages or discourages breaking appointments.

One of the basic tenets I teach dental practices is to make patients feel totally comfortable and welcome in the office. However, it is all right to lay a little guilt on those who thoughtlessly waste the doctor's or hygienist's time.

One reason for holes in the schedule is that staff members do not have enough hours in the week to complete all their behind-the-scenes chores—no organizational or "tooth fairy time." Therefore, subconsciously, receptionists are elated with a broken appointment. They know the clinical staff then will help with filing, confirming, ordering of supplies, organizing inventory, and working on recalls or collections. It is important that the front desk staff have the same motivations as the other team members for keeping cancellations to a minimum.

Another reason for a 15 to 30 percent production loss because of broken or canceled appointments is that there is no backup system for filling these holes the minute they occur. This deficiency is responsible for lost patients as well as big losses in production.

Pending Notebook

As a front desk person, I realized that I could not rely on my memory or the patients' good intentions to keep my appointment book filled. I also had another motive for designing a pending notebook: I knew my boss liked to stay busy with patients, but that when he didn't have one he came to the front desk to "help" me. That was motivating for me.

A pending notebook serves three valuable purposes and can add thousands of dollars to the office's annual production:

1. Patients will stop falling through the cracks of the appointment book.
2. The recorded information can be used to fill holes in the schedule the moment they happen.
3. A dental practice can be held legally responsible for "lost patients." This recorded information shows three attempts were made to reschedule—a big plus in the office's favor in the event of a "supervised neglect" case.

In a pending notebook, six tabs are purposely left blank because each office has four different major treatment areas. In general practices these areas may be "Crown and Bridge," "Root Canal Treatments," "Amalgams and Composites," and "Inlays and Onlays." In specialty practices the treatments differ, and tabs should be individually filled out. One of the six tabs is marked "Miscellaneous." The sixth tab is marked "Recall" and has leather-bound monthly dividers behind it.

The golden rule in appointment book control is "No patient should ever leave the office without his or her next appointment." If the patient's name does not go into the main appointment book, it is entered in a pending notebook under the type of treatment needed with the telephone number, treatment code, and length of treatment. Space should be left for comments.

Example 1:

If a patient who travels a lot leaves the treatment room needing a three-unit bridge, he may say, "I need to check my schedule at the office before making an appointment. *I'll call you.*" The receptionist should immediately turn to the crown and bridge section of her pending notebook and record the name, telephone number, length of treatment time, and treatment (in detail). This patient may leave the office, become extremely busy and forget to call. By listing the patient's name and proper scheduling information in a pending notebook, the nonappointed patient cannot slip through the cracks of the appointment book and become lost.

Example 2:

A mother calls the office and says, "My two sons have appointments tomorrow for fillings. I'd like to cancel those appointments because one son is ill." The receptionist automatically asks if she wishes to reschedule the time. If the mother says she doesn't know how long the illness will last and will call back, the receptionist turns directly to the Amalgams and Composites section of her pending notebook and writes the names of the two boys, telephone number, treatment code, and length of treatment time. These patients can be called if the mother forgets. Oftentimes, good intentions fall by the wayside, creating big losses in production and postponed treatments.

In one dental office in which I worked, I kept a Special Call List in the front of my pending notebook in order to fill last-minute cancellations and no shows. If patients lived or worked within a two-mile radius of the office, I did not reappoint them. If a patient needed a 40-minute appointment, I might say, "Doris, since you work next door at the insurance office, may I put you on my special call list and call on short notice?" Surprisingly, many of our patients said they enjoyed not knowing of their appointments in advance and liked being considered "special." Any time I had a last-minute change, I could count on finding someone to fill the space.

Train the entire staff not to use the word "cancellation" because no one wants a patient to know the practice ever has them. If a patient must be moved forward to fill space tomorrow, say, "We have a change in our schedule tomorrow at 3:00. Would you like to come in then?" If the word "cancellation" is used, the patient feels second best.

Tooth Fairy Time

Organization takes time and people power. The reason so many practices are disorganized is that staff members simply do not have enough hours in the week to get themselves organized, much less stay organized. More hours are not more production if you are not organized.

When does the clinical staff have time to properly clean and maintain the equipment, meet with sales representatives, or look through catalogs to compare prices of supplies? When do they have time to clean and stock the treatment rooms or the lab and to perform everyday housekeeping duties?

When does the business staff have time to call delinquent accounts, purge inactive files, and call patients not seen in the last year? When do they have time to call patients with large pending treatment plans, go over their insurance benefits, and set up future appointments and payment plans? When do they have time to clean and organize their work areas? Being organized starts with a clean environment.

If all these "tooth fairy chores" are done during production hours, the office is not reaching its full potential in terms of production. Offices that have adopted four hours per week of tooth fairy time have increased their daily productivity between $200 and $800. They also report happier office atmospheres and up to 10 percent reductions in overhead. Tooth fairy time works. Try it and watch the practice grow.

After beginning this "resurrection" of the practice with organizational tooth fairy time, an immediate change takes place in the attitude of the staff. The staff may tell the doctor, "I can do two days' work in four hours of uninterrupted time." Remember, happy staff are productive staff.

The practice begins to grow as the entire staff truly communicates with patients during patient time instead of doing the tooth fairy chores between patients. The doctor can schedule more patients in fewer hours because the patient has the staff's undivided attention during office hours.

A most welcome change occurs in overhead: it goes down. Nearly every expert preaches increased production. However, reductions in overhead also result in higher profits for the practice.

One office I visited spent $16,900 above the acceptable yearly average because they were farming out many things the staff could have done if they had tooth fairy time. This time can be the most productive four hours in the week.

Here are some examples of how savings were made in that practice. A $2,000 cleaning service was eliminated. Now the staff of seven does the weekly cleaning on their time as well as the daily cleaning. They divide the office into seven equal parts and create team spirit by sharing the housekeeping duties daily and weekly. All seven were in favor of saving this $2,000 annually as a means of increasing their own salaries and benefits.

The office saves $4,000 annually by eliminating a monthly accounting service. With a check-writing system, the business staff does the simple monthly bookkeeping, including accounts payable and payroll, and only needs a CPA report on a quarterly basis.

Almost $2,000 is saved annually by discontinuing a computer billing service. The office offers instant-billing (walk-out statements) and does not send statements for fees of less than $100 (lesser amounts are collected the day of service). Normally 60 to 70 percent of the statements offices mailed are unnecessary. They can be eliminated by requesting payment the day of service on noninsurance cases of less than $100.

By not using an outside collection agency, the practice saves thousands per year. The business staff has time to call delinquents and collect past-due accounts in the same friendly way that they deliver their dental care.

There also is a big savings in supply costs. A dental assistant has time to set up an inventory control that saves the office $200 to $400 per month through comparison shopping.

Saved overhead dollars should be spent to motivate the office with incentive bonuses and trips at the end of the year. Tooth fairy time is one of the best ways to help the dental team work together to provide quality dental care.

Time better spent is money earned. The better utilization of time by the dental team will add up to substantial savings for the practice. If these savings are translated to dollars, that amount of money becomes available for other needs. Set team goals for efficiency, and then enjoy the rewards. Stress will be one of the first factors to be reduced as the office becomes more efficient. When the stress level is dropped, office harmony increases. *The happy office is the more productive office.*

Chapter 6

Recall Systems and Purging

For years the recall system has been called the bread and butter of the dental practice. It is true that the healthier the recall system, the better the restorative practice.

This chapter addresses the problems in recall systems and tells how to improve the system the office is currently using. For offices that are not sure of their recall effectiveness, a simple formula for determining recall numbers is outlined.

Don't just presume bread-and-butter recalls. Like most good things, they have to be worked at and nurtured.

Is Your Recall Healthy?

Poor communication from office personnel to patients makes many dental recall systems fail or be less than effective. A recall system should be responsible for 40 to 45 percent of the restorative practice. Faulty recall systems have been the straw that broke the camel's back in some practices. Traditionally, doctors tend to panic when practice growth slows. Instead of evaluating the effectiveness of the recall system, they go in the other direction and try to cut expenses by reducing the number of hygienist days. This is nearly always the wrong decision.

Recall problems often center on conflicts between the doctor's and hygienist's schedules. Years ago most offices booked recalls six months in advance as a standard practice. That practice had the effect of locking-in the hygiene schedule.

If the doctor or hygienist wanted to take a day off, it was impossible because patients were already scheduled. Another problem of booking so far ahead was that the hygienist had difficulty seeing new patients because her schedule was full.

Yet another problem created by booking so far in advance was the resulting "holes" that appeared in the hygienist's schedule when the receptionist called to confirm the patients. Some patients had forgotten the appointment, others couldn't be reached, and many changed their appointments when they were contacted. Spending an hour or two daily trying to fill the holes in the hygiene schedule is a stressful activity for the front desk person.

Disillusionment with the system of booking ahead led to the era of "chase the recall cards" (send a reminder card and then chase it until an appointment is made). This job consumed up to 40 hours per month of business staff time yet was only up to 70 percent effective. Moreover, many patients fell through the cracks of this recall system. The money spent calling and recalling patients actually hurt rather than helped many practices.

Under this system many patients tried to postpone their follow-up care. Their response to a receptionist's call was often, "Has it been six months already? Let me check my schedule, and I will call you." If the receptionist tried again in another month, some patients began wondering if the doctor was having a problem. Was the fact that the receptionist had called more than once an indication that the dentist was desperate for patients?

Patients do not enjoy being hassled regarding follow-up care. Many think they are saving money by postponing recall appointments for several months. It is a public relations job for the dental team to educate patients that preventive maintenance is an investment, not an expense.

Booking ahead for recalls is a good technique. It is far less time-consuming than doing it all by telephone, and it increases effectiveness by up to 40 percent. By holding an hour open on the hygienist's schedule until a day ahead, new patients can be readily accommodated. With sufficient notice, most patients accept occasional reschedulings for doctor or hygienist needs. And appointment pre-confirmation cards sent in advance reduce the holes that appear when the receptionist makes the confirmation call the day before.

Recall systems are never completely effective, but some do border on the 95 percent effective rate. It's been said, "The mind is like a computer what goes in comes out in the form of action or reaction." If patient reaction to the recall method being used is not positive, then changing the system should be considered.

First determine how many days of recall your practice should have. A simple formula for determining recall days follows:

1. Count your active patients.
2. Multiply by 2 (as most patients are seen twice per year— some less, some more).
3. Divide by 12.
4. Divide by the number of days per month the office is open. This is the number of recalls daily.
5. To determine the number of hygienists needed, divide the daily recalls by the average number of patients per hygienist per day.

Example:

> 2,500 active patients × 2 = 5,000 recalls annually
>
> 5,000 ÷ by 12 months = about 416 recalls monthly
>
> 416 ÷ by 16 days — about 26 recalls daily
>
> 26 ÷ by 13 (average patients per hygienists per day) = 2 hygienists

Many offices have half the hygiene days they need and, as a result, they lose patients and experience low productivity. If your office does not effectively recall patients, someone else will.

Here are some communication tips to bring your recall system back to health:

Make the Recall Appointment TNT
(Today, Not Tomorrow)

The golden rule of patient retention is "No patient should leave the office without another appointment." The old advice

"Never book more than two weeks in advance" harmed many practices and sold tons of time-consuming recall systems for the companies advocating the phrase. A patient appointed in advance for three, six, nine, or twelve months is a committed patient—your patient.

The doctor and hygienist must choose their vacation time six months in advance and leave flexible time in the hygiene schedule (one day a month for continuing education, snow days, or illness). If the hygienist must have a day off for one of these reasons, the patients can be moved to the flexible date.

The amount of flexible time on a daily basis varies from office to office. In some ofices, changed appointments create flexible time. In others, one appointment per day is left open until 24 hours before the appointment (for new patients, those who need more than one appointment, etc.).

Hygiene appointments made in advance must be confirmed with a postcard that is mailed on the 25th of each month and is followed up by a phone call the day before. This TNT recall system has added thousands of dollars to the productivity of many offices, not to mention the hours of time it has saved for the staff by not having to chase recall cards.

Accept Your New System

Many offices say, "Our patients won't like booking ahead." As with any new system, if the dental team accepts it, the patients will. Proper communication creates enthusiasm for acceptance. The staff member should say, "If this time of day is good for you, Ms. Jones, let's reserve the same time in six months." (Always speak in an affirmative tone.) If the patient says she would rather have you call in six months, respond with, "If you schedule the appointment now, you'll have your choice of time and day. We know it's difficult to remember. That's why we confirm the appointment."

Review the Written Communication that the Office Mails to the Patients

Most of the recall postcards available on the market actually invite the patient to change or break the appointment. Many say, "If this time is *not* convenient, please call for another appointment." Others say, "This is to *remind* you of your checkup." The word "remind" annoys patients and may make them feel ignorant; "checkup" makes the appointment sound unimportant.

Get rid of those poor communicators. The wording of recall cards can help in keeping appointments. The following is a positive approach:

Dear Mr. Adams:

This is to verify the appointment you made with our hygienist for your dental cleaning and oral cancer examination. This time has been reserved just for you. Any change in this appointment affects many patients. We look forward to seeing you on _____ at _____.
                                                          (date)   (time)

Add the date and time of the appointment. The card should have been self-addressed by the patient in the hygiene room while X-rays were being processed or during post-treatment. A small clipboard can be kept nearby to hold the recall cards.

The follow-up care appointment is noted by the hygienist in a looseleaf appointment book kept at chairside. Hygienists should have their own one-column looseleaf appointment book (two columns for the hygienist-assistant team). When the appointment is scheduled, give the patient an appointment card and file the recall postcard in a January-to-December file box under the month the patient is due back. Keep the three- to twelve-month pages in the hygiene room. The current-to-three-months pages are kept at the front desk for confirming or occasionally for changing an appointment. On the 25th of the month prior to the scheduled recall appointment date, mail the self-addressed recall postcards to patients.

This process takes less than one minute, saves a dozen reappointments each day for the front desk person, and allows the hygienist complete control of her time to schedule the proper amount of time for each patient. Patients with less than a full dentition may not need the normal amount of time; difficult patients may need more.

Patients are much more receptive to scheduling their next appointment in a clinical setting with the hygienist than in a busy business office with its many distractions. When appointments are presented in a positive manner, patients are willing to book ahead.

Give the recall system a checkup. If it is causing stress with too many no shows, changed appointments, and wasted hygiene time, these changes in communication with the patient will help improve the percentages. Treating the reappointment as an important health-related event rather than just a checkup encourages patients to keep their appointments.

Get Floating Recalls Back on the Book

There is a sleeping giant in most dental office filing systems. Purging records effectively can reap gold from those files. There are thousands of dental dollars in patient records just waiting to be tapped. Knowing how to get these floating recalls back on the appointment book can add income and bring the peace of mind that patients are no longer being lost.

Not many years ago, purging patient records was a rather haphazard procedure in most dental offices. Records were pulled when the filing space was exhausted. Staff members then removed the charts of patients who had moved or died. That was all there was to it.

In the early sixties, "purging the files" was added to the dental management vocabulary, and it became a more standardized, although time-consuming, procedure. Each patient's record was examined to review the date of the last visit, a chore that often took months of staff members' time. Once purged, these inactive files were alphabetized, placed in cardboard boxes, and stored. Occasionally a former patient would reappear, and an inactive file was retrieved and reactivated.

In the seventies, filing systems became more efficient. With the use of year stickers, or purging labels, to indicate the year of the patient's last treatment, the task of purging charts now takes minutes rather than months. At the end of a calendar year, say 1986, the secretary simply pulls all records with labels prior to and including 1985. The number of records purged depends, of course, on the patient load, number of years in practice, and how transient a population the practice serves.

In most dental offices, the business staff adds the year sticker before filing the charts for the day. If the office is a busy one, however, the stickers may be forgotten. I usually recommend having a box of year stickers in the treatment rooms. As the patient's bib goes on, so should the year sticker on the chart.

Many dental offices take advantage of these simplified purging procedures but continue to place inactive records in a storage area. If your office is guilty of this, it may be losing out on thousands of dental dollars! These inactive patients, or floating recalls, can provide an easily accessible pool of patients to boost production.

How can inactives best be returned to the practice as active patients? Contacting them by mail produces a 25 to 35 percent response. That approach incurs, of course, the expenses of printing, postage, and secretarial time. A telephone campaign, perhaps conducted when the doctor is away from the office, results in a much higher percentage of reappointed patients.

It is essential that the staff member making these calls sound caring and enthusiastic. The reappointing success is proportional to how goal-oriented the staff member is. The purging person must be chosen with care.

If the practice is in an area with a stable population, a reappointment rate up to 65 percent may be expected using the following telephone conversation when contacting inactive patients:

```
Good morning, Mr. Johnson. This is Linda from
Dr. Wilson's office. We are updating our pa-
tient records for the current year. Your last
appointment with Dr. Wilson was September
16. Because your follow-up care is very im-
portant to our office, would you like to make
an appointment at this time or be placed in
our inactive patient file?
```

No one wants to be taken out of the active files if they have any intention of ever returning. Using the above conversation, you will encourage a good percentage of the patients contacted to be back on the book that day.

Although an ultimatum may sound harsh, it encourages patients to reschedule and brings better results than any previously tested method. No patient wants to be considered "inactive;" it may mean the doctor will be unavailable for emergency treatment or that the patient may be treated differently on the next visit.

If the patient intends to return and has been postponing the next recall appointment, the ultimatum brings the appointment decision to the surface and compels a response.

If the patient says, "Go ahead and place me in your inactive files," this normally means he or she is seeing another dentist. Most patients will not call to offer this information, however. The staff member then should say, "Oh, Mr. Johnson, we are sorry we won't be seeing you and your family on a regular basis. Please keep in mind that a telephone call from you is all that is necessary to have you back in our active files." By saying this, you have communicated that it is okay to visit another dental office, but also that the patient will be welcomed back to your practice.

Negative feedback from patients can be extremely valuable. Many doctors and staff never know why they've lost patients. The reactivation call is an excellent time to try to extract reasons for dissatisfaction from these patients. To get the valuable information needed (to sound thorough, not nosy), the staff member should say, "To complete our records, may I please chart the reason you wish to be inactive?"

The patient almost always will give the staff member the true reason. Common complaints expressed by patients are an uncaring attitude on the part of doctors and staff or being kept waiting too long.

Sometimes a patient identifies a previously unknown problem such as (1) "I was never pleased with the shade of my crown," (2) "I was kept waiting too long," (3) "My treatment plan was not fully discussed before treatment," or (4) "My child's problems didn't seem important to anyone there." In such an event, offer the "problem" patients a free consultation appointment to smooth the ruffled feathers and to discuss the problem. Many of these hidden problems are rectified easily, and the patients become good missionaries because of the office's desire to satisfy its patients.

Remember: Patients don't care how much you know until they know how much you care.

After a reactivation call is completed, the staff member should write down the name of the patient, whether appointed or not, and, if inactivated, the reasons for the patient leaving the practice. The purging person also should give a report at the monthly staff meeting . An example, "Last month, in purging, I called 67 patients. Of these, 43 made appointments, 3 left for [this reason], two left for [that reason]," and so on. Both doctors and staff need to know why patients are being lost in order to correct any problems that exist.

After that invitation and display of caring by touching base, many patients return because they know the office is concerned about them.

Touching base annually with lost recalls increases productivity by a large percent. Productivity also may be increased if the receptionist engages in some public relations as a part of the purging process. If a patient makes an appointment for recall, the receptionist should invite other family members who may also be overdue for an appointment or are not currently seeing a dentist. "Invite" is the key word to doubling new patient referrals.

To create more enthusiasm in this purging job, divide the purged patient records evenly among the staff. Team members might receive $1 for every patient they successfully reappoint in their purging calls. An incentive bonus of $2 could be given to team members for every new patient booked through a family member called.

In order to have current names and addresses on file, the hygienist should fill out a self-adhesive label with the patient's current name, address, and telephone number at the time of treatment. As she updates the patient's medical history, she can also update the patient's personal profile. The label should be clipped to the chart at chairside and then placed on the ledger card or added to the computer data when it reaches the business office. If ledger cards are copied as a billing procedure, the information so obtained should be typed on each ledger.

If the patients' files have not been properly purged, start today. Only by doing this on an annual basis can an effective recall system be maintained. Reactivate the inactive patients—within every practice lies another partially dead practice that is awaiting a personal call. Efficiently updating the patient records can contribute greatly to an increase in production. With a minimum of work by all staff members, each patient can be tracked and reappointed.

By having a healthy, active recall and purging records annually, the office should be busier than ever with nonstop increases in production. Even though it should be the patients' responsibility to take care of their oral health, they do, in fact, look to the dental team to help them preserve a healthy smile through follow-up care. If your office doesn't follow through with patients, another office may have the opportunity to provide their dental needs.

Chapter 7

Inventory
Systems

In dental practices, few items of overhead expense are controllable. Rent, utilities, and staff salaries cannot be easily reduced. But it is possible to exercise some control over the dollars that are expended for supplies. Most offices order their business and dental supplies haphazardly, often wasting thousands of dollars per year. These offices could become wise shoppers and, with the money saved, treat the entire office to a seminar or exciting vacation. Money saved and so invested improves morale and skills and ultimately increases the overall production.

Business Supplies

Most dental offices lack storage space to sufficiently control their business inventory. When the business supplies are stashed here and there in drawers or cabinets or anywhere else space is available, it is difficult to know what is on hand. This lack of organization is extremely costly because it results in overordering or underordering.

The best storage situation for business supplies is a walk-in closet with open access shelves. In some offices I recommend using the enclosed shelves of the built-in bookcase filing system as storage for paper products if the separate storage closet is not available.

Cluster all similar paper products together such as patient information forms, stationery, envelopes, and marketing materials. Time is wasted ordering paper and business products if the supplier has not been documented at the last purchase. If someone has to spend a few hours looking through catalogs to find a particular product or form, time has been wasted. And time is money.

Remove all paper wrappers and boxes from the business supplies (except envelopes). Place one sample envelope over the end of the box to show what style envelope is in the box.

Fold 3″ × 5″ index file cards or business cards in half to make reorder tabs for stacked paper products. On the lower half of the back of the folded card, type the item name, stock number, place of purchase, telephone number, quantity ordered, and price of the last purchase. Place the reorder tabs at the two-month supply level in each stack of printed material.

When the materials reach the two-month level, pull the reorder tab and place the order for the item. This simple system of organizing the business supply inventory eliminates the problems of trying to remember where to order products and of over- or underordering.

When you need to redesign your new patient information form, print a quarterly patient newsletter, or "welcome to our office" brochure. Find the best price by calling two or three printers. The first step in printing is to determine the needs such as quantity, quality of paper, color, and size. Get bids from the printers and ask for a breakdown in prices by quantity. Printed products drop drastically in price per unit with higher quantities. The fewer ordered, the more per piece. The cost for 1,000 units usually is little more than for 500. Always ask for the prices of larger quantities. If the product is one that will remain the same, buy the larger number. If it is a dated item or you expect it to change soon, order a smaller quantity.

Only one business staff member should be in charge of ordering business supplies. The person so designated should be a wise shopper who enjoys finding good deals. A good rule of thumb is this: staff members should spend the office's money as they would spend their own. I know of dental offices that annually spend $3,000 to $5,000 more on supplies than they should because the staff members in charge are not conscientious shoppers. Staff members who continually save the office money through careful shopping should be openly appreciated.

Dental Supplies

An effective inventory control system for dental supplies saves both money and stress. As with the business supply area, proper storage is the first step toward efficiency. I highly recommend open-shelf, lateral storage for easy access and visual control. If supplies are stashed in out-of-the-way places such as under cabinets, in drawers, and in several rooms, it is difficult to be efficient.

The central supply area can be a small room or walk-in closet with shelves at an accessible level. Bulk storage items such as paper towels, toilet tissue, and patient towels should be kept on higher shelves. The more frequently used items should be at eye level or lower.

Inventory bins keep hard-to-stack items neat on the shelf and aid in the rotation of products for maximum shelf life.

The bins come in all sizes and materials and can be ordered through a wholesale paper products or dental materials dealer. The most popular bins are made of corrugated cardboard. They are high on the sides and back and low in front. Use a magic marker to list the contents on the end of the bin. Before ordering a supply of inventory bins, measure the shelves and determine the various widths needed.

Rotating dental supplies can save money and assure that all products are fresh. It is tempting to put fresh items on the front of the shelves as they are being unpacked and to take the front items off the shelf as they are needed. Consequently, there's the peril that the products at the back of the shelf will never be used. Always move old stock forward. If you use the inventory bins when restocking, lift the bin off the shelf, move all materials to the front, and restock the back of the bin with fresh supplies. This is especially important with products that have a limited shelf life.

Ordering four times per year in bulk is an efficient use of time and it saves money. Offices that order bimonthly usually pay top dollar. Many doctors are reluctant to pay rent on the storage space that would allow them to have their own minimum-level dental supply store on hand. Yet the additional money spent by ordering frequently could pay the storage space rent many times over and minimize interruptions for the staff member who places the orders.

Some dental supply companies offer storage of bulk rate items at no additional cost to the doctors. They give coupons for a year's supply of the product. When the doctors need that particular item, they send in the coupon for delivery of the product. This works well for an office that wants to save money by ordering in bulk but has limited storage space. Other dental supply companies offer a free inventory system in exchange for the office's exclusive business. Many dental offices that use this system report their supply costs are at a comfortable level and their staff members' time is being used more efficiently.

Good supply representatives can be very valuable to a practice. Many offices, however, swear by the mail ordering method of acquiring supplies. There is no right or wrong way in this regard.

It's been my experience that those dental practices which stress quality care and service to their patients are the same offices which appreciate the value of good supply representatives. These professional sales representatives are service-oriented; they offer more than just products. In fact, the ones I know act as consultants to the offices they serve. They offer loaner equipment, trial products, and fast repair service. Good advice is this: Get a good sales representative and stick with that person. The nickels you save on mail order may not be worth the dollars you lose if you have an equipment malfunction. I believe in saving money where possible, but don't give up the services that sales representatives can provide without carefully examining the decision.

Dental supply costs should be 5 to 7 percent of the gross if the office has an efficient system. Check the percentage monthly by having the assistant in charge of dental supplies divide the total dental supply costs by the total collected for the month. This figure should be discussed at the monthly health-of-the-practice staff meeting (see Chapter 3). Depreciation items such as equipment are not part of the average.

Years ago, to keep track of supplies, suppliers, and orders, we used recipe file cards and had an alphabetized card for each product ordered. The problem with this system was that we spent a lot of time looking for the filed card. With two-by-two's, for example, should the card be filed under T for "two-by-two's," G for gauze squares, or J for Johnson & Johnson?

To address this problem, I developed a color-coded inventory control system that works very well in all offices. If this area of your practice needs reorganization, the system will help. In general practices, I recommend categorizing the products into nine groups:

1. Operative and surgery
2. Cotton and paper products
3. X-ray and prophy materials
4. Anesthetic and needles
5. Lab and impression materials
6. Cleaning and sterilizing
7. Endodontic supplies
8. Burs and diamonds
9. Miscellaneous

A tracking system is set up by making an inventory card for each item used. The cards are then divided into the nine categories and held in a visible record notebook for easy accessibility.

The system comes with colored dots and strips, so the indexes are color-coded. As an example, if hygiene products have a red dot, all hygiene supplies are stored on the shelves with red tape or labels and any cabinets that house hygiene products have a red dot. Color coding is easy and saves time looking for items.

The inventory system should be controlled by only one clinical staff member. It is like the appointment book: when more than one person writes in it, there are problems. The system lists the centrally supplied items only. As items are received and checked on the shipping invoice, write it in the inventory control system under "received."

Double-check the item's quoted price to be sure the billing department picked up on any specials quoted by the sales representative. Also check the unit price times the quantity to confirm the multiplication. Add each invoice twice to make sure the totals are correct. Place a red check mark on the invoice by the date received and file it in the monthly order folder in chronological order.

At the end of each month when the bills are received, the assistant in charge of dental supplies should check each invoice number and price against the field invoices for the month. Then she should clip them together if correct, write "correct," initial them, and place them in the accounts payable folder for payment.

Many dental offices lose hundreds of dollars because they pay invoices as received. Honest mistakes can happen. Double check every invoice before payment is made. The money saved is worth the time spent in verification. Laboratory cases should be handled in the same manner. Some dental offices have paid twice for the same case because they did not double check.

A "Want List" and "Back-Order List" should be posted in the laboratory or storage area. When anyone on the staff notices that the office is about to run out of a particular item, it should be everyone's responsibility to write the item on the Want List. Many offices keep reordering back-ordered items. Then when the back orders start coming in, the office has enough of the product to last for years. Two metal tabs (different colors) can indicate "on order" or "back order." When an item is ordered, place a colored tab on the inventory card (Fig. 7-1). Put the second color tab on the card for back-ordered items to prevent their being reordered.

The dental office should set goals to keep controllable expenses low. A little time spent on organizational work can save money and frustration. Decide now where the office will go in a year on the saved amount. The enthusiasm and excitement created among the staff by a continuing education course or fun vacation will repay the investment many times over through increased office production.

DATE ORDERED	DATE RECEIVED	QUANTITY ORDERED	QUOTED PRICE	IN	OUT	BALANCE ON HAND

Item/Stock #

Supplier

Phone #

MIN_____MAX_____

Fig. 7–1   Sample inventory card

Chapter 8

Collections

Collecting fees in the same friendly manner in which the dental care was delivered is an art any dental team can develop. It requires a positive attitude coupled with excellent communication skills. It also is necessary for the doctor to cooperate by allowing the business staff to enforce established policies.

This chapter addresses the step-by-step collections process from formulating policies to administrating past-due accounts. Many offices do not have set payment policies. This causes confusion at the front desk and obstructs cash flow. Other offices have such policies, but the person at the front desk is handicapped in executing them because of the intervention of the doctor.

One of the biggest causes of an escalating accounts receivable is what I call the "Dr. Nice Guy" syndrome. Patients frequently say, "Doctor, I really want to have this treatment we just discussed, but I don't know how I'm going to afford it."

Too often the doctor then says, "No problem. I am sure we can work something out." In essence, the doctor is saying, "Money is the least of my concerns. In fact, I don't even care if you pay me." And, as we all know, that simply is not so.

Doctors usually should not be involved in *how* patients are to take care of their fees. If they do, a barrier is set up between the business staff and the patients. In such instances, patients tend to resent the business assistant's attempts to enforce office policy. When Dr. Nice Guy is kept out of such conversations, the accounts receivable get smaller.

104

When a patient looks to the doctor for forgiveness of payments, the response should be, "My business assistant Betty handles all our payment arrangements. I am certain the two of you can work something out." It is unfair to the business assistant for the doctor to side with patients who are not complying with office policies. The business assistant is the one who must deal with these patients in the future; she is also the one who is blamed when patients get behind as a result of Dr. Nice Guy's intervention. The clinical staff can best assist the business staff by saying to patients (as their charts are handed to them at the conclusion of appointments), "Please give this to Betty at the front desk so she can write your receipt for today," or "so Betty can process your insurance forms immediately."

Realistically, I do not believe a dental office can operate successfully on a strict cash-only basis. However, up to a 98 percent annual collection rate is possible with a few realistic expectations and some know-how. About 95 percent of dental patients can be expected to pay on time, about 3 percent pay sooner or later, and about 2 percent never pay. Remember that both individuals and practices tend to get out of things exactly what they expect. The dental office that expects a big collection ratio is seldom, if ever, disappointed.

Collection Philosophy

In establishing payment policies, I recommend that the entire dental team jointly discuss the subject and then, after decisions have been made, commit them to writing. Written collection policies ensure that both staff and patients are informed and that the administration is consistent. All the staff must be aware of the guidelines. If staff members are confused or uncertain, they will project this feeling to the patients. Although actual collections are the responsibility of the business staff, all staff members should be able to converse intelligently with patients about payment policies.

Collection Philosophy
The old adage that honey attracts more flies than vinegar is true in collecting past-due dental accounts. The philosophy should be to inform before you perform, to communicate with

patients about fees and payment arrangements, and to never surprise a patient in regard to fees.

Collection Goal

The goals should be to keep accounts receivable at a comfortable level (no more than 1.5 times the monthly production figure) and to keep the accounts up-to-date through good policies and follow-up. If you have a lower than 90 percent collection ratio one month, strive for a more than 100 percent collection the following month. Good collection ratios for the year are 95 to 98 percent.

Collection Policy on New Patients

Cash, check, credit card, or insurance should be required at all first visits. This information is given to each new patient over the telephone on initial contact.

Collection Policy on Lab Cases

Half should be collected on the preparation date and the balance on delivery or half on the preparation date and the balance in three equal monthly payments, with the first due on delivery date.

Collection Policy on Insurance Patients

The deductible should be collected on the first visit and any out-of-pocket portions as treatment progresses. On large insurance cases, half the out-of-pocket portion should be collected on the preparation date and the balance on delivery or half the out-of-pocket portion on the preparation date and the balance in three equal monthly payments, with the first due on delivery date.

Collection Policy on Treatments Under and Over $100

For treatment fees of $100 or less, payment should be collected on the day of service. A credit card may be used to provide more than the normal cash or check service. For fees more than $100, payment options should be available through your bookkeeping department.

Fig. 8–1 is a sample form for suggested payment options. This sheet should be in duplicate form. The first signature is that of the patient, and the second signature is that of the responsible party (if different from patient).

Doctor's Name and Address

PAYMENT ARRANGEMENTS

Patient Name _____

Address _____

City _____ State ____ Zip Code _____

Home Phone No. _____ Work No. _____

I choose the following method of payment for dental care performed for myself and my immediate family.

I. I Have No Dental Insurance

A. I elect to pay cash ____, check ____, Master Card ____, or Visa ____ on all visits as treatment progresses.
B. I prefer to secure a bank or other loan for the entire amount of the treatment and will make monthly payments to the lending institution.
C. On extensive treatment, I elect to pay 50 percent on the preparation date and the balance in three equal monthly payments.

II. I Have Dental Insurance. (_____)
(Company Name)

A. I elect to pay my deductible of $ ____ and any out-of-pocket portion on the preparation date (due to lab fees and other expenses) and the balance on completion or delivery date (normally three to four weeks later).
B. On extensive treatment, I elect to pay 50 percent of my out-of-pocket portion on the preparation date (due to lab fees and other expenses) and the balance on completion or delivery date (normally three to four weeks later).
C. On extensive treatment, I elect to pay 50 percent of my out-of-pocket portion on the preparation date and the balance in three equal monthly payments.

Signed _____   _____
            Patient   Responsible party

Date _____

Fig. 8-1 Sample payment options form

In establishing payment arrangements, use the above as a guideline and add any other options (see below) that may be indicated for the practice. Patients need concise knowledge of treatment and payment plans. Remember, be candid: to surprise a patient is to lose a patient!

Criteria for Granting Credit

Become a member of the Retail Merchants Association and local credit bureau. Before granting any credit over $ ___, check the patient's credit worthiness by calling one or both of these organizations.

Interest Charges

Interest or finance charges may be added to all cash accounts after 30 days at 1.5 percent of the unpaid balance. Insurance accounts may have the same amount of interest added to all out-of-pocket portions after 30 days of receipt of the insurance check.

Note: Be aware that you must notify all patients in writing at least 30 days before the office begins charging interest if it has not done so in the past. Also, on interest accounts, all patients with four or more payments must sign a truth in lending agreement (Fig. 8–2) outlining the payment arrangements. Print a truth in lending agreement form in duplicate on office letterhead and give a copy to the patient.

Patient _____ Person responsible _____

Address _____ City _____

State ____ Zip code _____ Phone _____

Description of services to be rendered:

Approximate number of appointments _____

1. Fee for services
   $ _____

2. Down payment
   $ _____

Fig. 8–2 Federal truth in lending agreement

3. Amount financed

   $ _____

4. Finance charge _____ percent

   ₵ _____

5. Total payment due (3 plus 4)

   $ _____

6. Total charges (1 plus 4)

   $ _____

The amount listed as "Total Payment Due" is payable to _____ at the above office address in _____ monthly installments of $ _____. The first installment is due on _____ 19____, and each subsequent payment is payable on the same day of each consecutive month until paid in full.

In the event the account should become delinquent for a period of 30 days, I hereby acknowledge that I will be responsible for all the balance, interest, and court costs and/or attorney fees.

I hereby certify that I have read and received a copy of the foregoing disclosure statement this _____ day of _____, 19____.

Signature _____

Fig. 8–2   Federal truth in lending agreement *(Cont'd.)*

Statement Date

Mail all statements on the 15th of each month and make delinquent account calls 10 days later on or near the 25th of each month or mail A–M statements on the 10th and N–Z statements on the 25th to keep the office cash flow even. Make delinquent account calls on or near the 20th and the 5th of each month, 10 days after the statement sections are mailed.

Information to Secure a Bank Loan

If patients find the half-down policy on larger cases a burden, instruct them to secure a bank or credit union loan. The lending institution can loan the entire amount, and the patients then are able to complete their dental treatment while making smaller monthly payments over an extended period of time.

Note: How do consumers buy cars, trucks, boats, homes, furniture, and other desired items? By using credit. This is what banks are for—to loan money to those who need it. Dentists who have stopped trying to be lending institutions find their practices operate more smoothly and with better control.

Credit Card Information

Display the Visa and Master Card logo in your business office, and mention credit cards throughout your payment option conversations and in presenting fees. Many people prefer to use "plastic money" and write one check per month for their miscellaneous expenses.

Credit card vouchers are mailed to the bank within three working days. All charges exceeding a certain amount must be approved with a verification code number by calling the toll-free credit card number as the transacton is taking place. (Patients may have exceeded their line of credit limits, so get verification immediately.)

Bookkeeper's Allowance

Do not refer to any courtesy or allowance as a "discount" because the term is inappropriate in a health-care setting. Offer a 5 percent bookkeeper's allowance on all fees over $300 if paid in full by cash or by check at the initial visit. Also offer senior citizen courtesies to all patients over age 65.

Presentation of Fees

All fees for each day's visit should be presented to each patient on dismissal. Always use positive terms for positive results. Refrain from asking, "Would you like to pay today?" or "How would you like to pay?" Instead, first reappoint the patient; then say, "Your fee for today's visit is $[amount]. Will that be cash, check, or credit card?"

Insurance patients should be presented the fee as usual after reappointment, but the presentation should be "Your fee for today's visit is $[amount]. We will be filing your insurance form immediately. Your approximate portion is $[amount]. Will that be cash, check, or credit card?"

Another situation might be when a patient's treatment is $1,000, insurance coverage is $700, and the patient's portion is

$300. Say, "Mr. Wilson, your insurance company will be covering approximately $700 of the $1,000 fee. Your portion will be approximately $300. Half your portion ($150) will be due at your next visit, and the balance upon completion of treatment."

These sample payment policies should be used as guidelines in the establishment of policies that fit the doctor's and office's philosophy. Remember, patients will be as lax in their payments as the office is in setting and enforcing payment policies. Firm office policies result in lower accounts receivable.

Enforcing Policies

To help patients accept the payment policies, the staff needs to know how to handle various situations that may arise when patients try to get around policies. Training staff to use specific solutions will give each person on staff the confidence needed to handle such situations. The following are a few situations in which patients want to make exceptions to the practice's policy guidelines.

Example 1:

A patient has a $500 balance which is due on delivery of a three-unit bridge. What if, on the day the bridge is to be cemented, the patient says on the way out, "Something came up. I don't have the money. Please bill me."

Solution: *Before* the patient is seated, the front desk person should say, "Oh, Ms. Smith. You are early for your appointment. Come on back to the business office so I can write your receipt for today." Hopefully, the patient will be early and have the payment as promised, and the bridge will fit!

Example 2:

A patient has very good insurance—80 percent on restorative—but all five family members need extensive dentistry. The 20 percent for which the patient is responsible could build quickly during treatment and pose a financial problem later.

Solution: The business assistant can speak with the financially responsible person and say, "Mr. Jones, your insurance coverage is very good—approximately 80 percent of the usual, normal, and customary fee. However, because all your family members need extensive treatment, your portion could be rather significant. The last thing we want to do is create a financial burden for you. Many families in this situation find it helpful to pay small amounts of $25 each visit as treatment progresses to lessen the amount due at the completion of treatment." Most patients appreciate such concern in not overburdening them financially.

Example 3:

A new patient needs restorative treatment totaling $1,500. Although the patient has no insurance coverage and no available cash, she reports that she has good credit.

Solution: The dental staff member should say, "Ms. Peters, because we are on a cash basis with our laboratory, our office policy on extensive treatment is half down on the first visit and the balance on completion of treatment, which is usually three or four weeks later. Rather than create a financial burden for you and your family, we would like to suggest an option that many of our patients choose. They find they are more comfortable securing a bank or credit union loan for the entire amount and then making small monthly payments over an extended period. We find that bank and credit union loans are easy to secure for dental purposes." The benefit of this approach is that the office will have a cashier's check for the entire amount on the preparation date and the patient will be able to handle small monthly bank payments. If the

office offers a 5 percent bookkeeper's allowance on fees over $300 that are paid in full by
cashier's check on the first visit, this option
becomes even more attractive.

If the patient questions the policy, say, "if we become a
lending institution, Ms. Peters, our dental fees will have to be
considerably higher to cover the costs of administering such
accounts."

If a patient states that his or her spouse gets paid next
Friday and asks to send a check, say, "Do you have your
checkbook with you? We will be happy to take a check dated for
today and hold it until next Friday."

For the patient who has forgotten a checkbook and does not
have a credit card, say, "That is fine, Ms. Miller, we will be
happy to give you a walkout statement (pegboard receipt if on a
pegboard system) and a stamped, self-addressed envelope so
you may drop the check in the mail when you get home."

If prior payment arrangements have been made and the
patient does not have the agreed-upon payment at the end of
the first preparation appointment, say, "Mr. Walker, I am sure
we discussed your obligation for today's payment. As you
know, we are on a cash basis with our laboratory. Therefore, we
will not be able to send your case to the lab until you have met
this obligation."

Changing Payment Policies

If a practice has been a billing practice, this does not mean it
must always do so. It is never too late to change office policies.
Many dentists are apprehensive about changing their payment
policies—afraid of offending patients by the change. There is
some justification to such misgivings. If a policy change is not
handled with tact, some patients may be lost.

First, the change must show there is a benefit for the
patient, not just the office. Second, the change cannot be
abrupt. And third, the change must be communicated properly.

For example, suppose an office that has always billed hires
a new business staff person who is experienced at presenting
and collecting fees assertively at the front desk. The new
business staff member should discuss with the doctor the

advantages of changing the payment policies. The member must know if the doctor wants to change and, if so, explain how the changes can take place without alienating the patients.

Another example might be that of a young dentist who has purchased an existing practice that has huge accounts receivable and "spoiled" patients. The young practitioner must talk to all team members to identify the problem, offer the remedy discussed below, and then ask for the staff's assistance in implementing change. To make an abrupt change in either example could result in stress and lost patients.

After determining what the new office policies will be and committing them to writing and rehearsing them, a positive letter should be sent to each patient of record. The policy change should include what, where, why, when, and how. The change should go into effect 90 days from the date of the letter to avoid abruptness.

The letter shown in Fig. 8–3 can be used as a guideline in developing a change in policy.

Dear _____,

Effective _____ our office must make a change in policy regarding payment of accounts. This change is necessary due to the increased cost of postage and bookkeeping services. Making this change will assist us in keeping our fees as low as possible.

Beginning _____, fees less than $100 will be due when services are rendered. We offer Visa and Master Card for your convenience.

For fees in excess of $100, payment arrangements may be made in advance through our bookkeeping department. We offer a 5 percent bookkeeper's allowance on all fees over $300 if paid in full by cash or cashier's check on the day of treatment.

Insurance deductibles or percentage of fees not covered by dental insurance are due when services are rendered.

We appreciate your support in our need to make this change in the provision of dental care for you, our valued patient.

Sincerely,
[Signed by dentist]

Fig. 8–3 Sample change in policy letter

If the doctor and staff believe in the policies, the patients will accept them.

Collecting Past-Due Accounts

Before making collection calls or offering extended payment plans, the dentist and staff must be aware of three major federal regulations. If staff members are not aware of these regulations, they can inadvertently jeopardize the practice. If the dentist uses a collection agency that does not abide by these laws, the *dentist* can be held liable. A copy of these acts can be obtained through your local credit bureau.

All staff making collection calls should abide by the Fair Debt Collections Practice Act that took effect in 1978. Excerpts of this act include the following:

1. Never make libelous statements. Never state or imply that, because of nonpayment of debt, a debtor is dishonest or a cheat. Never make a baseless threat of criminal prosecution.
2. Never harass the debtor or his or her family by making repeated telephone calls. Calls after 9:00 P.M. and prior to 8:00 A.M. (in the debtor's time zone), on Sundays, on legal holidays, during periods of religious observance, and other times prohibited by local legislation are forbidden.
3. Never use extortion. Never make threats to distribute negative credit information to an association or to communicate with the debtor's employer. Do not contact anyone directly or indirectly, except the debtor, regarding the past-due account. On a joint account, the debtor's spouse may be contacted.
4. Never use profane, obscene, or abusive language. Never touch or even hint at physical action. You can be sued for actual or implied assault and battery.
5. The law prohibits the collector from falsely implying he or she is working for a government agency.

Outside of personal contacts, the telephone is the most effective method to collect payments—seven times more effec tive than collection letters. The caller must be well versed in collection tactics to be effective. If you follow the suggested conversation, keep a positive attitude, and remain within the restrictions of the law, accounts receivable will not be a problem. These calls are designed to make both the staff member and patient feel comfortable while reducing the accounts receivable.

Listed below are characteristics of a professional collection call:

1. Never lose control.
2. Never hang up first. Be courteous.
3. Enunciate clearly.
4. Use strategic pauses.
5. Always establish a definite payment arrangement before ending the conversation. Get two verbal agreements during the conversation: the date the payment will be received and the amount of the payment.
6. Always make a written record of what transpired.
7. Never argue about money.
8. Be consistent.
9. Keep a positive attitude. It is important to feel you are performing a valuable service for the office. If you do not feel comfortable making collection calls, someone else in the office should be assigned this task.

Determining when an account is delinquent and when to make the first past-due call is important. The calling should begin 15 days after the payment due date or 45 days after the treatment date if no payments have been made. I recommend pulling all ledger cards (if you are on a manual system) or underlining in red on the computer analysis report those patients who should receive a delinquent call.

The calls should be made at a time when the collections person can devote adequate uninterrupted time to the task. Try to reach the patient at home first. Remember that the information regarding the balance cannot be discussed with anyone except the person responsible for the account or that person's spouse, if a joint account.

The call should be firm, polite, and to the point. "Hello. Ms. Webber, this is Joan from Dr. Wood's office. I am calling in regard to your outstanding balance of $150. We haven't received a payment since March 3. There must be a problem." In stating that "there must be a problem," the staff member gives the patient an opportunity to offer an explanation in a nondefensive manner.

At this point the collector should be sympathetic to the problem the patient presents and then continue with "I am very sorry you have been out of work. However, our accountant was in last week to review the accounts. He will be back next week for a report. May I please tell him what day of each month you will send a payment and the amount of that payment?"

Note: I find that using an outside "ghost" of an accountant removes the "bad guy" image from the office and makes the conversation more comfortable for the patient and staff person. As Zig Ziglar says, "You shouldn't tell a lie, but you can tell the truth in advance." If the accounts are not kept up-to-date, the accountant *will* ask why.

Let's suppose the patient's response is "My husband handles all our finances, and I cannot give you the date or an amount."

The staff response should be this: "That is fine Ms. Webber. Please discuss it with him tonight. I will call back tomorrow for your answer."

If the patient becomes threatening or argumentative, the collection person should end the conversation with, "I obviously caught you at a bad time. Perhaps you would rather call me at a better time."

Calling patients at their place of business can become a liability situation for the doctor if the call is not handled properly. The collector cannot say anything to the patient or spouse at work that might produce embarrassment in front of co-workers. In rare cases the debtor may claim defamation of character.

To be on the safe side, if the office must call patients at work, make sure proper phrases are used. An example would be as follows: "Hello, Mr. Wells. This is Alice from Dr. Rolen's office. We need to discuss your past-due balance. If this is not a comfortable time for you, please return my call before 5 P.M. today." In asking the patient to return the call, the collector is providing the opportunity to avoid embarrassment in front of co-workers. Patients appreciate this act of consideration.

A second-month call is necessary whether the patient pays as promised or fails promise to pay. An example of the second month's call for paying patients would be as follows: "Hello, Mr. Wells. This is Alice from Dr. Rolen's office. I am calling to thank you for your $50 payment, which we received on January 12. We will expect the same amount by the 12th of next month and appreciate your cooperation in clearing the account." The delinquent patient should be called monthly until the balance is paid. When the calls stop, often the payments do, too.

Kindness and empathy are necessary in successful collection campaigns. I have actually made "friends" with patients I called each month. If patients have temporary financial problems, it is always the "nice" collectors who get paid first when their finances improve.

If the patient says he or she will send $40 on the 15th of each month, make a note of this. These verbal agreements should be documented in the collections system on the patient's alphabetized information page under "Comments" (See Fig. 8–4). The patient's name and telephone number and the amount should also be recorded behind day 15 in a 1 to 31 tickler system (days of the month). (See Fig. 8–5.)

The collection calls are made monthly from A to Z. The 1 to 31 tickler system should be checked daily for unpaid promises. For example, on the 18th of the month, check back three numbers to day 15. Look at the promise-to-pay sheet. If the $40 payment promised on that date beside the patient's name has not been checked off, the person should have a second call that month. "Mr. White, this is Jenny from Dr. Black's office. The payment of $40 you promised on the 15th has not been received, and today is the 18th. If it is not in the mail already, I would appreciate it if you would bring it by the office or place it in today's mail."

Name _____

Home Phone _____   Work Phone _____

Date of first call _____   Amount Due _____ Date of last payment _____

Comments: _____

_____

_____

Date of second call _____ Amount due _____ Date of last payment _____

Comments: _____

_____

_____

Date of third call _____ Amount due _____ Date of last payment _____

Comments: _____

_____

_____

Date of fourth call _____ Amount due _____ Date of last payment _____

Comments: _____

_____

_____

Fig. 8-4 Alphabetized patient information sheet for collections

A few patients give repeated, unkept promises that waste time and create stress for the collection person. After several attempts produce only empty promises, I recommend sending the patient a final notice. This can be a form notice or a letter from an attorney or a collection agency.

Collection agencies are not recommended because they keep a large percentage of what they collect. And attorneys usually only handle large accounts. If the office systematically keeps its accounts under control, outside services are not necessary.

MONTH	NAME	PHONE #	TO PAY

Fig. 8–5 Sample promise to pay form

Small Claims Court is a last-ditch effort that can be made after a final notice. In some states small claims are profitable to the small business owner; in other states, where garnishment of wages is not allowed, small claims tend to be a waste of time. Getting a judgment in states that allow garnishment of debtor's wages carries clout for the creditor. Some employees can lose their jobs if their employer is named in a small claims dispute.

If the office decides to go the small claims route, the court must have a correct address in order to serve the patient the notice. There are a few tactics you may want to use to locate a patient's new address. The new patient form can be a valuable source. Ask the question, "Nearest neighbor to contact in case of an emergency." A neighbor is more inclined to tell you where the patient is working or living than a relative is. To request a forwarding address, you can send $1 to the claims and inquiry office of the post office. Include a self-addressed, stamped envelope and the patient's name and last address. You also can use third-class mail. Send an envelope to the patient's last known address and mark it, "If forwarded to new address, notify sender on Form 3578. Postage for notice guaranteed." If the patient has moved and sold the family home, send a letter addressed to "Occupant." Request that the new owner send the patient's address on an enclosed, self-addressed postcard.

If you have the correct address, it is not necessary to have an attorney file for you. Any staff member can learn to perform this task. Small claims procedures vary from place to place. Call your local magistrate for information pertaining to your area. Listed below is information you may need to compile your claim:

1. Location and hours of the Small Claims Court.
2. Whether applications to submit to the debtor can be mailed to you or must be picked up at the courthouse.
3. Other forms that need to be completed before or after the court date.
4. What information should be taken to court.
5. How much notice the debtor needs between the court date and the date the warrant is received.
6. The court fees.
7. Where the docket (list of cases for the day) is located. (You may need to record the line and case number for the judge.)

The purpose of the small claims suit is to obtain a judgment that will order payment or permit garnishment of the patient's salary or attachment of his or her assets. Again, state laws on collections vary. Call the civil division of the local district court and ask your questions.

The longer an account is delinquent, the less chance the office has of collecting. Most offices could take their entire staff on a vacation on the money lost to noncollectibles, to outside collection services, and in unnecessary monthly statements.

As Dr. Omer Reed stated at the 1985 American Dental Association convention in San Francisco, "People who owe you money don't like you." Start making patients like your office. Set firm yet acceptable payment policies, allow the staff to enforce the policies, and get collection calls going on a consistent, monthly schedule. Remember, firm office policies result in low accounts receivable.

Chapter 9

Insurance

Negative attitudes about dental insurance can destroy practice productivity. Many staff members and even some doctors regard insurance as a nightmare of paperwork and more bother than it is worth. Such attitudes can gravely handicap an office. On the other hand, if the office develops a positive attitude about insurance, the referrals may double. A simplified insurance system can turn the paperwork chore into a challenge.

Third-party payment or dental insurance has swept the profession with many pluses and a few minuses. Changes occur almost daily in the insurance business. They will continue to occur as new plans, such as direct reimbursement and PPOs are evolved.

Insurance Attitudes

In the beginning, dental insurance plans were vehicles for reimbursing patients for what they had spent on dentistry. However, dentists soon caught on that insurance payments could be looked upon as assured accounts receivable. These dentists began to realize that if they accepted assignment of benefits and allowed the insurance checks to come directly to them, they were simplifying the process for their insured patients. This started the practice of copayment—patients paying only their part of the fee and the office waiting for the insurance check.

Dental insurance provides four important pluses:

1. Dentists are able to provide higher-quality dentistry, not just the "drill 'em, fill 'em, and bill 'em" variety.
2. It improves patients' knowledge of procedures.
3. It increases referrals from each place of employment.
4. It adds additional gross income to the practice.

As patients became aware of dental insurance and the value of this benefit, there began to be a few frustrations in the dental offices that were providing the services.

Many employees were told by their employers, "This form is your passport to free and complete dentistry. Take it to any dentist, and the doctor will even fill it out!" At that point, it became the job of the dental staff to smile and say how happy they were the patient had this wonderful benefit, but that the insurance was only a partial payment. After their deductible had been paid, they also were responsible for any balances after insurance. Insurance plans are benefits (super aids) but not the free rides many employers imply.

Patients need to be informed that the care, skill, and judgment that produces optimum dentistry sometimes costs more than the insurance company's usual and customary fee. One of my patients said it well. I was almost apologizing to her for a dental fee not being covered at the percentage she had expected. Her response was, "I wouldn't go to a dime store looking for a wedding dress, nor would I seek out the cheapest dentist in town—I want the best." I realized then that people feel about their teeth the way they feel about other important purchases: "I only want to go through this once. I am not that concerned about the money, just make it right!"

The response for dentists who have "shoppers" in their chairs is "Let's do it right, not do it over. You have a mouthful of patchwork dentistry. I only do for my patients what I would do for members of my family." Stress quality and that you offer it. Remember if you don't believe in yourself, no one else will. It isn't just a matter of selling yourself. The office must believe in quality and that its patients deserve nothing but the best.

With dental insurance, patients must understand the office policies on paying their portion. The deductible should be paid on the first visit, and any out-of-pocket portions should be paid as treatment progresses. On large cases, patients should pay half their out-of-pocket portions on the preparation date and the balance on completion of treatment or in three equal monthly payments. (Clear up long payment arrangements, and broken appointments will clear up simultaneously—they go hand in hand.)

With large preauthorized insurance cases, set up the preparation appointment in four to six weeks and the payment arrangements for the out-of-pocket portion. You can have loosely defined, not detailed, arrangements such as: "Ms. Stewart, your plan normally pays 50 percent of usual and customary fees on crowns and bridges. Because we use *better-than-average* dental labs and materials, our fee may be higher than the allotted average fee. Your portion could be approximately $600 of the $1,000 estimate. Our normal arrangement is to have the patient pay $300 when we start and the remainder when the crowns are delivered." Always go for the most favorable arrangement initially. The half down and three equal monthly payments plan can be offered as a secondary alternative if necessary.

It amazes me how many dentists and their staff unknowingly talk patients out of treatment by saying things like, "Let's send your preauthorization off and see how much the insurance company will pay." No wonder patients don't get the dentistry they need: the doctor or staff have programmed them to believe they can't afford the balance.

Remember that most people don't know what services they need, so start programming your patients to want what the office can deliver—quality dentistry. A better comment in the above example would be, "Ms. Stewart, you are so lucky to have an insurance plan to pay a portion of your care. Let's make the appointment for six weeks. By then the form will be back, and you will have made arrangements for the $300 down payment. You are going to be so happy with the end result of a healthy, beautiful smile."

It's important that patients sense the staff's enthusiasm for the proposed dentistry. One of the reasons there is so much incomplete dentistry is that no one in the dental office was enthused about the prospective result.

In selling anything, you must stress the "What's in it for me?" angle. Therefore, a sales approach will vary with the personality and emotional needs of the individual patient. If you can identify the different personality types of your patients, you can decide what type of approach will be best to take in your communications with them.

If you are dealing with achievers, give them the facts. Don't waste their time. Even though they are leaders in their fields, they are impatient by nature. They make good politicians because they make things happen. They are the implementors.

If you are dealing with a patient who influences others, you need to realize that you are talking with someone who is a social, talkative, outgoing person. For such people, their greatest need is for social approval. Talk about beauty and social advantages to them.

The steadfast, loyal, hard-working patients are the easiest to deal with. Their only fault is that they sometimes can resist change. They are the patients who "think about" their treatment the longest but like the change the most once it has been done. They will promote you to others.

Another personality group is the compliant patient. These people are perfectionists to the maximum. They want lots of explanations and are hard to please. They trust you the least. But if you please them, they will send their friends and relatives.

Being able to read people is a must in selling and dealing with patients. Understanding how different people react can assist the staff in their interactions with the public. If the dental team realizes that the same approach does not work on everyone, they can tailor their presentations.

Patients who walk out of the office after accepting treatment recommendations and while awaiting the preauthorization answer sometimes get "buyer's remorse" and cancel the plans for the treatment. With a future commitment (another appointment and payment arrangements), they are much more apt to proceed with the treatment. It is imperative that schedules be made and that the patient understand the benefits involved in having the dentistry completed.

One of my clients had a problem with long appointments being canceled the day before because the patients didn't have the out-of-pocket portion that was due. This created stress for the receptionist in filling the canceled time on such short notice. This office now has an arrangement whereby the half down is due seven days prior to the appointment. The patient is given an addressed, stamped envelope for mailing the retainer fee. For this practice, the policy works like a charm. Again, if we believe in our policies, our patients accept them.

If the office is not familiar with a particular insurance plan, ask the patient to bring the insurance booklet on the next visit. I recommend that each office compile an insurance reference card system for each treatment room to enhance the communication and marketing skills of staff members. These are $3'' \times 5''$ index cards on a large, silver ring that hangs inside a cabinet door near the dental chair. The cards are filed on the ring alphabetically by employer's name (the company that employs the patient). Listed are the following:

Company name
Insurance carrier name
Telephone number
Deductible amount
Percentages paid on various treatments
Maximum for year

For example, I am a patient in the dental chair and say to the assistant or hygienist, "Judy, I really need to have that bridge done—approximately how much would be covered by my insurance?"

It doesn't work too well if Judy says, "I don't know. Rita is our insurance person, but she is here only on Tuesdays and Thursdays. You will have to call and ask her." Not only does that response give the office a look of incompetency, it loses tons of business each year. Some staff do not know; some do not want to know. Winners will compile the insurance reference cards and will appreciate the availability of the additional information. Losers will say, "That's not my job" or "I don't know and don't care to know."

By keeping a set of insurance reference cards at chairside in each treatment room and another at the front desk, everyone in the office becomes knowledgeable. For instance, the assistant,

Judy, could pull the cards and say to the patient, "Let's see, you work for Piedmont Airlines. According to our latest information, it looks like they will pay approximately 50 percent of your treatment."

Or the doctor may be alone in the office seeing an emergency patient on a Saturday or Sunday. The truck driver says, "I have dental insurance. But if they don't cover the root canal, pull the tooth." The doctor whips out the card file, looks up Ryder Trucks, and says, "According to our latest information, your insurance covers approximately 80 percent of all restorative, including endodontics."

"Great, let's save the tooth!" he replies. Caring and being informed go hand in hand.

When talking about insurance, always use the word "approximately," Patients tune in on numbers. Never say the insurance company will pay a certain amount; do say, "according to our latest information" and "approximately."

Major medical claims should be filed in all accident cases. If the patient has an accident that results in crown and bridge work, always file major medical, as it normally pays 80 percent on crown and bridge. With large accident cases under major medical, I recommend calling the insurance representative before treatment because some plans have obscure clauses.

In drawn-out accident cases involving litigation, the office can and should apply for up-front money to cover lab and other expenses. It is simply a matter of writing to the attorney and making a request. The attorney files an advance expense form. If nothing is requested, the office may wait months or even years for a settlement. Most attorneys are cooperative with such requests. It is certainly worth the time to file a request.

With large accident cases, turn lemons into lemonade by doing all you can to support the case. One dentist I know takes photos of the trauma site, medical treatment, and post operative results. He always sends the attorney representing his patient copies of the photos and treatment progress reports for which he charges $75 to $125. This doctor is now recommended by the State Bar Association to handle big accident cases because he knows how to make attorneys look good in court.

As my friend Zig Ziglar says, "You get out of life what you want when you help others get what they want. You can't help someone else without helping yourself."

"Coordination of benefits" means husband and wife both have insurance coverage. Until 1984 the husband's plan was always considered primary for his treatment and for all of the family's children. The wife's plan was primary for her treatment only. In 1984 some insurance carriers said it was discrimination and inequitable for the husband's plan always to be the primary carrier. With the 1984 law, the parent whose birthday comes first in the calendar year is the primary carrier for the children and the other parent is the secondary carrier.

Insurance Processing Simplified

Some dental offices do not accept assignment of insurance benefits on the patient's first visit. Other offices do not accept assignment at all. Those practices that do not accept assignment of insurance benefits lose patients by that decision. Patients go down the street to another dentist who does accept assignment in order to avoid having to pay insurance-covered costs in advance.

Everyday insurance handling can be a breeze if the office is efficiently organized. Some staff insist on making dental insurance a chore, but it can be simple with the right attitude and daily follow-through.

There should be no backlog of dental insurance in any office. This is sloppy bookkeeping and puts a crunch on the office cash flow. Computerized insurance is nice for efficiency, but the quick claim works wonderfully well, too. Some call the quick claim a "super bill." I don't recommend that terminology because some patients think "super bill" means "big bill."

With a quick claim form that fits a pegboard, insurance can be processed manually just as fast as if it were computerized. The quick claim is a triplicate, preprinted insurance form listing all the treatments and code numbers. The doctor's name, address, and Social Security number are also preprinted, which saves the insurance clerk about eight hours a week in an average solo practice. This form is attached to the insurance form the patient fills out (employee portion) and signs.

The quick claim should be designed by each doctor and staff to fit their particular clinical needs. Spend time designing just the right form. The representative from the pegboard system can help. Ask the representative for copies of other dentists' forms to serve as idea sources for the design. After deciding on the design, I recommend ordering the minimum number the first time in case additions or deletions are subsequently desired.

Using the quick claim is really quite simple. The patient's name, previous balance, and quick claim form number are logged in on the pegboard as the patient is registered. The quick claim goes to the treatment room with the patient record after the numbered form is logged in. The clinical staff circles or underlines the treatment performed today, and fills in the teeth numbers and surfaces while the information is fresh in their minds. (All code numbers are preprinted.) When the form comes back to the receptionist, it is three-fourths completed. The clinical staff or doctor also writes what will be done and the time needed for the next appointment at the bottom of the quick claim. It doesn't matter who writes in the fees. In some offices, the clinical staff member does; in other offices, the business assistant fills in the fees. The quick claim is checked at the desk; then fees are totaled and posted on the pegboard after the patient is reappointed.

The patient receives a copy of the form that will be submitted that day. The second copy is attached to the insurance form the patient filled out and signed, and the top copy is filed in an "insurance pending" tickler system on top of the desk. This is a rack of 13 file folders marked January through December and one for preauthorization. File the office copy of the pending insurance form alphabetically in the month folder in which it is mailed. For instance, all insurance forms that leave the office in February are filed alphabetically in the February folder.

The office copy is pulled when the insurance checks are posted. The paid insurance forms now go into an A to Z clutter file in a drawer or a box under the desk—never in the patient's chart.

At the end of March, go through the February folder. If four office copies remain, this alerts the staff that four insurance payments are past due. I recommend calling these four patients and having them do their own insurance inquiry. Insurance companies act fast when the subscriber yells. (When the dental office yells, so what?)

The conversation to the overdue insurance payment patient is, "Ms. Jones, this is Linda from Dr. Brown's office. We mailed your insurance claim in the amount of $78 on February 12. It is now the end of March, and the insurance check has not been received. It is our office policy to wait a maximum of 60 days for *all* insurance checks. In two weeks, if the insurance check has not been received, we will ask that you pay the $78. If and when the insurance company sends a check, we will be happy to reimburse you." Getting the patient involved brings immediate results in most cases. When the irate subscriber calls, the insurance company reacts.

This insurance tickler system is simple and effective. The bookkeeper won't have to spend hours going through the accounts, trying to determine which ones are past due. Check the preauthorizations weekly. Don't be afraid to call or write the insurance companies if they take too long to respond on preauthorizations.

To simplify the manual insurance handling further, try these time-saving tips:

1. On a copier, run several copies of the patients' insurance forms after they have filled out the employee portion. Ninety-five percent of the insurance companies will accept a clear, duplicated copy of the employee's insurance form with a quick claim attached. (Be sure to white-out the date and signature before the forms are copied.) Always request a fresh patient signature and current date on the photocopied form.

2. To eliminate wasted time in addressing insurance envelopes with the lengthy insurance company addresses, I recommend taking a box of 500 blank No. 10 envelopes to the printer with the five major insurance companies' addresses pasted on the center of five envelopes. Cut out and paste the doctor's return address or logo on the upper left-hand corner of the same five envelopes. Have 100 envelopes printed for each of these frequently used companies. Preaddressed insurance envelopes can save up to 20 minutes daily.

At the end of the day, if the insurance has been properly handled on each transaction, it should take no more than five minutes to get the insurance forms in the mail for the day. Take all the insurance forms with completed quick claims attached out of the insurance basket. Sort the forms by insurance company, and mail all those going to the same company in one envelope. If X-rays are requested, do not send originals. Use a duplicating machine or double film. The original X-ray should always be part of the clinical record.

Some offices hire an insurance person to work on insurance forms all day long. This is a waste of time and money in most offices. The completion of an insurance form should be a team effort with everyone doing a share to simplify the task.

Letting the insurance pile up to be done a day or week later is as inefficient as allowing each patient to leave the office unappointed. Remember the phrase "Do it now!" Anything placed aside to do later takes two to three times longer to do because we must reprogram our thoughts back to the original procedure. Having an outsider come in to do the task later takes even longer because this person is unfamiliar with the circumstances.

Turn your insurance chore into an insurance challenge with a team approach and a sensible follow-through insurance system. Each job in the dental office is as difficult as everyone makes it. Remember, today's insurance patient is tomorrow's assured accounts receivable and everyone's next paycheck.

Chapter 10

Team Approach to Marketing

Marketing of the dental practice (internal and external) has become fashionable today. Many staunch traditional dentists who once vowed that "I built my practice on quality dentistry and that is all I will ever do" are now wondering where many of their patients have gone.

Patients leave practices for various reasons such as moving away, dislike of staff, lack of attention, and quality of care. One thing is certain: patients like to feel special. When new doctors open practices, they have time to make their patients feel just that way—special. But no matter how long the doctor has been practicing, the entire dental team should try to make all patients feel that same way: new-patient special. Doctors and staff often commit the mistake of spending extra time and effort making new patients welcome while treating their returning patients as just so many warm bodies in the chairs.

New Patient Numbers

The entire dental team must be aware of the need for healthy new-patient numbers. This figure should become part of the annual goal-setting and monthly monitor for the practice. Some offices feel they have a healthy number of new patients at 12 per month. Other offices have no idea how many new patients they have monthly because they don't keep score.

Many offices fail to realize that new-patient numbers play a significant role in determining a practice's success.

A practice in the $250,000 to $400,000 range must have 25 to 40 new patients (including emergencies) per doctor to maintain that level of production. Pediatric practices need to double the number to 50 to 80 per month for the $250,000 to $400,000 practice.

To determine whether you have a healthy new patient load, do these simple calculations. In an average practice:

    25 new patients monthly = $250,000/year
    30 new patients monthly = $300,000/year
    40 new patients monthly = $400,000/year
    50 new patients monthly = $500,000/year

In pediatric practices, double the new-patient numbers.

Some practices bill $300,000 annually but see 45 to 50 new patients monthly. They are underproducing $150,000 to $200,000 annually. On the other hand, some practices see only 25 new patients monthly yet produce over $400,000 annually. They may be overselling or using high fee schedules, or they may be exceptionally efficient in handling patients and are therefore producing more per month for the number of patients they see.

Emergency Patients are Great Practice-Builders

If a new patient expresses discomfort on the first call, the staff should treat that patient exceptionally well. Emergency patients can become enthusiastic missionaries for the practice if they are well cared for on their initial visit. Many staff (and some doctors) view emergencies as interruptions, bad-paying patients, and general nuisances. The truth, nearly, is that the office can be losing thousands of dollars annually by turning away emergencies or giving them second-class treatment. As noted earlier, it has been estimated that a well-treated emergency patient is worth approximately $1,000 a year in continued care and referrals.

While giving an after-dinner lecture one evening, I made the statement about the value of emergency patients. An older dentist interrupted to say, "Ma'am, I hate to dispute our distinguished speaker, but emergency patients in my office aren't worth $25. In fact, they don't even pay their $25 extraction fee."

Later that same evening, another doctor came up to see me and said, "Linda, don't ever stop preaching how important emergency patients are. Just a month ago, I had an opportunity to see two of that doctor's patients. One case is over $4,000 and the other is about $2,000. If he doesn't send another patient for six years, we are still ahead of your statistics."

Emergency patients can be examined, X-rayed, anesthetized, and then returned to the reception room while the scheduled patients are seen on time. After the emergency patient's immediate discomfort has been relieved with an anesthetic, he or she should be content to wait until an opening develops in the scheduled. Many offices get the emergency patient in the chair and do not know when to stop treatment. This is an unacceptable practice if scheduled patients are being kept waiting.

Proper Staffing for Emergencies

In order to build a practice by treating emergency patients, the office must be properly staffed and equipped. The ideal situation for the average solo practitioner is one auxiliary for each dental chair. The minimum number of chairs should be three, but four or five are even better. Some dentists say a new room of equipment is too expensive to install. The question that needs to be asked is how much the new room and chair will return on your investment. If the answer is $100,000 per year, the investment is wise. If the chair will sit idle half the day, the investment is poor.

Many dentists and staff fool themselves with scheduling. In some offices with two assistants, a full-time hygienist, and one or two front desk people, I could easily condense what they schedule in a five-day week into three very productive days. Because dentists often view staff as overhead, they limit their full potential by being understaffed. If the office is in fact understaffed, it will underproduce.

Always remember that staff members are investments, not overhead. If properly trained and utilized, auxiliaries produce for the practice three to seven times their salaries. Emergency patients cannot be used as practice-builders with two few staff members. Watch attitudes toward emergencies change from negative to positive when the office is properly staffed to treat them.

Involving the Staff

No matter what internal or external marketing the office chooses to implement, the staff should always be involved. They will develop much more enthusiasm for making ideas work if they've helped create them. I recommend trying at least one new marketing idea each quarter—several if they are closely related.

Example:

Improve the reception area for the patients' comfort. Under this one idea could come several ideas for change:

1. Improve the quality of reading material. (As we know, the caliber of reading materials suggests the educational level you feel your patients have.)
2. Place nicely bound cookbooks in the room along with recipe cards imprinted with the doctor's logo, address, and telephone number at the top. Patients that wait can copy the recipes they like.
3. Add plants and small containers of potpourri to the reception room to give it life and a pleasant fragrance.

Offices that do not try new ideas become stale and humdrum. Patients will respond to the innovations, and this should determine which ideas work and which are not so effective. Give new ideas at least a six-month trial. You cannot do everything you learn at seminars or from books. Replace old ideas with new ones for variety.

It also is wise to seek staff input in gift-giving at holiday time (especially for the specialty practices that send gifts to referring doctors). Try to be unique. The entire dental team should look for gift ideas all year. Craft shows often have clever gifts that can be personalized for the people on the list. Gifts purchased at the last minute to beat a holiday deadline are least effective.

Dressing for Success

Proper attire in the dental office is as much a part of the marketing package as anything else. Image is important to any business. What statement does your office want to make to its visitors?

Some doctors have the misconception that they shouldn't look too successful because patients may think they charge too much. Therefore, they do not dress well. Such a belief can have a negative effect on the practice. Dressing poorly not only turns off the quality patients who are sensitive to details but also creates a low self image.

Self-image is directly reflected in office fee schedules. I can tell a doctor's level of self-image when I review the fee schedule. Poor self-image and low fees go hand in hand. If you want to be successful, you must look successful. Start working on radiating pride.

Staff attire and grooming are also important parts of the office success statement. I always can tell a sharp office when I meet the staff: they look sharp.

Tips on Developing a Positive Inward Self-Image

1. You can't love anyone else until you love yourself.
2. You will become the person you think you are.
3. Self-image starts with a feeling of self-worth and importance.
4. You will become what you "hang out" with. Surround yourself with others who have positive self-images.

Dressing to Develop a Positive Outer Image

How we dress is a statement we make about ourselves to the world. Are you confident and outgoing or shy and introverted? A new wardrobe, accessories, or uniform will make you feel good about yourself. Others will treat you exactly the way you treat yourself.

I often am asked what the dental team should wear in the office. There are no set rules. Several factors dictate the office dress code, such as (1) the geographic location of the office, (2) the age of the doctor and staff, and (3) the age and type of the majority of the patients.

A dental office in Chicago or New York may be differently attired than a practice in Oklahoma or Texas.

In a golfing community, dental professionals can get by with casual attire during office hours. In a downtown location, however, patients may wonder if the doctor would rather be golfing than treating patients. In rural practices, where patients may wear bibbed overalls and flannel shirts, office attire should be less formal than the shirt and tie worn in most urban offices. Some midwestern practice staff wear tasteful jeans to the office. These offices report that the patients enjoy seeing the staff in Western wear because most of the patients dress the same. But if all the patients came dressed in business attire, they would feel the office is much too casual in jeans and probably would seek a practice with a more professional look.

Some people wonder why age has anything to do with office attire. More mature dentists prefer the conservative uniform look, while younger professionals tend to be less firm in dress codes for staff and more relaxed in their own dress.

If the practice has mostly elderly patients, the dental team must dress fairly conservatively because a casual appearance will be a turn-off. Business people will expect a serious and professional appearance for the dental team. However, farmers and ranchers may feel uncomfortable if the office is too formal. Children easily identify with the dental team that wears t-shirts and casual attire. When in doubt about the mode of dress, look at the patients and the sales representatives who call on the office. Sales people normally dress appropriately for the business look of the region.

Regardless of location and type of practice, I strongly feel that the more successful you look, the more successful you become. The dental team needs to establish a common ground with the patients so everyone feels comfortable and confident.

The following is a list of suggestions for successful dressing:

Suggestions for Clinical Staff

1. Polished, white clinic shoes
2. Coordinating fabrics in different styles most flattering to each figure type
3. Conservative makeup, professional hairstyles, simple jewelry, and perfume in moderation

Suggestions for Business Staff

1. Business attire, such as blouses and blazers with skirts or slacks
2. Well-groomed hair, makeup, and nails
3. Stockings and business shoes (not spiked heels or sandals)
4. Tasteful jewelry and accessories

Suggestions for Dentists

Male

1. Dress shirt and tie, dress slacks, and quality leather shoes
2. If a smock is worn chairside, make sure it is in good taste and impeccably pressed and cleaned. No polyester—they went out of style in the seventies. Blends such as cotton, linen look, and quality synthetic fabrics are an up-to-date look
3. A sports coat or dress jacket when out of the office in public, unless at casual affairs

Female

1. Quality suits, blouses, dresses, and accessories with a business/professional look
2. Quality leather shoes, stockings, and a handbag for a matched ensemble
3. Makeup and grooming in good taste with a professional look
4. Quality lab coat (if worn chairside)

Dress codes for the entire staff office should be outlined in the office manual to avoid misunderstandings.

If the office offers a uniform and grooming allowance, spell out the expected use of this additional income. Doctors who provide this benefit want to see their investment properly used.

Office Appearance and Ambience

One of the most overlooked areas of marketing in dentistry is the appearance of the entire office. Some reception rooms are so outdated and worn that many patients have been lost to more modern and well-kept offices. Patients judge the unknown (dentistry) by the known (the appearance of the office and its surroundings).

The clinical areas of some offices still use old equipment. Even at its shiny best, it gives the office a look of despair. Patients see the equipment or the way the doctor dresses and think, "If he is 15 years behind in the equipment or the way he dresses, I wonder if he is 15 years behind in the dentistry."

The modern dental office should not reflect the starched professionalism of the past. Today's practices need to be warm, friendly places that patients enjoy visiting. Adults as well as children need to feel welcome the minute they walk through the door. If children use the practice, make an effort to have something in the reception area that appeals to them. A rocking chair and a teddy bear convey to the child that he or she is welcome and expected there.

Public relations such as this cannot be bought with money. If the child is happy, the parents are happy and tell their friends. The word gets around town fast. Cater to children, and see what happens to the adult practice. Internal marketing such as this is beyond value.

Incidentally, the receptionist's best public relations will be hampered if the business office has outdated features such as a frosted window and a sign that reads, "Please ring the bell and be seated." How impersonal! Worse yet is a sign-in sheet. This belongs in the military. Patients resent it, and half of them forget to sign.

Sign-in sheets are only indicated for practices such as ortho, which see 40 or more patients daily. If the office must use a bell, at least have a sign that reads, "Please ring the bell, so we may say hello." "Please ring the bell and be seated" essentially says, "Sit down and shut up."

If you are too busy to be nice, you are understaffed. If you must have a glass window, make it clear glass. The receptionist needs to be able to see the entire reception area. If she is on the telephone when the patient arrives, she can always smile and nod. It is best to have the receptionist in an open setting so there are no barriers between her and the patients. The frosted glass could appear to be hiding something—especially to children. If the receptionist has visual access to the patients, she appears more friendly.

The patient's bathroom should be the most beautifully decorated room in the office—at least as nice as the guest bathroom of a home. It amazes me how many practices still have the institutional towel box with white or brown scratchy paper towels for the patients' use. Would you have these in the guest bath at home? A "community terrycloth towel" is not the answer, but how about soft, pastel paper towels on a wooden dispenser?

I also recommend wallpaper, carpeting on the floor, paintings or pictures, silk flowers, or other decorative items. For the patients' comfort, there should be mouthwash samples, disposable toothbrushes, and floss. A tray of hand location, hairspray, and colognes add a welcome touch. Some readers probably will say, "Is she kidding? Our patients would walk off with these niceties!" If that happens, perhaps you can have a basket of disposable items on the receptionist's counter.

Cleanliness

As important as keeping the office aesthetically pleasing is having the office spotlessly clean. The pride we have in our personal surroundings reflects the pride we have in the work we do. Everyone can and should share in an effort to have a shining, clean office.

It amazes me how some people can work in a dirty office and never see how it really looks. The office should be dusted and vacuumed daily, sinks should be polished at all times, and trash receptacles should never be within view of the patient. I have heard patients say, "I judge the sterility of the instruments by how clean and tidy the entire office is." Would your office pass the patient test?

A patient once left a practice because the same dirty cotton roll was on the floor in front of the sink two weeks in a row. She decided, appropriately, that they did not clean very thoroughly.

All staff and doctors should sit in the dental chairs and the reception room at least once per week and look around. In a reclined position in the dental chair, do you see bugs in the light or ceiling tiles that need to be replaced? In the reception room, do you see dust on picture frames, chipped paint on wood-work, and outdated, torn magazines? Patients may not know for years how great your dentistry is, but they immediately know how they feel in your office. The little things you do make the big impression.

Location and Signs

The outer appearance of the office, the street location, the sign on the street or building, and the facility itself are the first impressions patients receive about the practice. If the building is attractive and the location is good, potential patients will note this. When they need a dentist, they will remember, "I liked the looks of that dental office on Maple Street, and it is close to work." The attractiveness of the building can have a major marketing impact on the practice.

When selecting the office location keep in mind that a dental office is much like a restaurant. Three things are impor-tant to success: location, exposure, and area. Dental offices in second-class areas rarely attract first-class patients. Practices located in industrial areas usually serve workers from nearby plants. If a shopping center is selected, most patients will be the ones who shop at the mall rather than at specialty shops or discount centers. In short, location includes the caliber of the clientele. It's important for dentists to know which types of patients they want to attract when selecting the office location.

Exposure is essential to practice success. Highly traveled areas with good street exposure bring the best new-patient results. Years ago a dentist could be successful with little exposure. As a matter of fact, some did not even have a sign indicating where the office was located. Not to have a sign in today's climate is professional suicide.

The exterior sign on the building should reflect the quality of dentistry being offered. It is the office's calling card on the street. The sign should match the building in design. For instance, contemporary offices need a contemporary sign, traditional offices need a traditional sign, and colonial offices need a colonial sign.

Dentists' signs should have an identifying statement depicting the type of dentistry provided. Before being erected, signs should be evaluated by the ethics committee of the local dental society. Before advertising became permissible, the ethics codes were stringent. Today, they are less strict; but there is merit, nonetheless, in seeking approval of the sign before its construction. Some municipalities have codes regarding signs and their design. Building owners also want some say in the appearance of outside areas. Check with each of these before investing in the sign.

In the sixties, general dentistry was in vogue. In the seventies, the theme was family dentistry. Neither of these labels is a good identity statement today. General is too general, and family is a practice-killer in the eighties. Cosmetic dentistry is the theme for today. Patients who need complete rehabilitation and those interested in cosmetics tend to be in the over-40 age group.

Dentists who identify their practice as "family dentistry" are hurting their cosmetic business because the message excludes many patients. As an example, when our two children were young, we did everything as a family and patronized family businesses. Now that the children are grown, we go out of our way to avoid family businesses. It isn't that we don't like children, it is just that we are more comfortable doing business in adult places.

The term "family dentistry" may cause some single patients to exclude themselves on the presumption they must be married and have children to be a patient. This is a growing sector of the population and one that controls much disposable income. (One family dentist reported that some of his patients thought the entire dental staff was a related family!)

If the sign on the practice does not depict the identity statement desired, change it. Be sure the office is conveying the correct message to the public.

Logos and Business Cards

Quality in this area is essential. Everything printed that leaves the office is a direct reflection on the quality of the dentistry. The office stationery and business cards should be tasteful and distinctive if such an image is a practice goal.

Hire a graphic artist to draw a logo, or give the assignment to an advertising agency. An agency will conduct research to determine whether the logo is similar to any others. The extra expense of using an agency brings the peace of mind of knowing your logo is clear of possible infringements. Simply hiring a graphic artist is cheaper initially; but if you have to change logos because someone else's is similar, the final expense is considerably greater.

The type of paper, ink, and printing used in business cards and stationery is very important. Raised lettering and more than one color costs more, but the result stands out as true class in a pile of letters or a handful of business cards.

Classic bond is good paper for stationery and envelopes. The linen look is very tasteful. And an embossed logo on the letterhead or business card adds a special touch.

No matter what type of paper is chosen, in logo marketing, simplicity and class are the keys. Cuteness in marketing was overdone in the dental profession in the late seventies. Logos with a dentist on ski toothbrushes do not present a professional image. Patients may say, "Isn't that cute?" but they really think that dentistry is a serious business, at least as far as they are concerned. They often wonder, "Does he take his dentistry more seriously than this fun card?"

The "Gentle Dental Care" and the "We Cater to Cowards" slogans were great until they were overdone. A patient or two may say, "I came because I saw the slogan in the Yellow Pages." Great, but does the practice want all the cowards? And there's the peril that the secure patients may say, "No wonder the doctor never sees me on time. He's treating all those cowards."

Yellow Pages

The controversy of whether to display advertising in the Yellow Pages is a big issue these days. Many doctors use Yellow Pages advertising very successfully. There are others, of course, who will never change from the one-line listing in the phone directory. But there is a middle-of-the-road approach that is both ethical and productive.

Dentists who use big Yellow Pages ads do get more new patients monthly. Dentists who are ultraconservative in their listings do not stand out in the Yellow Pages. Their new-patient numbers come from referrals, not from the listing. There is nothing wrong with patient-referred patients—they're usually the best. But by not having any Yellow Pages referrals, the office can lose up to 30 percent of the new patients that a more significant listing would produce.

I do not advocate big ads. I do feel, however, that bold print within a thin line encompassing the listing is a plus. It is easy to locate, makes a professional identification statement, and is always in good taste.

Doctors who use bold advertising with success should continue the campaign. We should only change those things that are not working. If the practice provides quality care in a professional, clean environment and has a caring staff and doctor, it normally will be strong regardless of how much advertising is done.

When in doubt about whether to advertise, ask these questions:

1. Is this our philosophy — Is it us?
2. Will I feel as comfortable with my colleagues? (Does that even matter?)
3. If I were the patient, would I select this dentist based on the ads?

If the answer to any of these questions is "No," revamp the advertising until everyone is comfortable with it.

Giveaways

Marketing in dental practices usually includes giveaways. Giving selected, appropriate items to patients is a nice way of thanking them for coming.

Pediatric practices often give away balloons, bravery badges, and other toys. Children are always thrilled with gifts.

Parents are pleased, too. The giveaways are usually inexpensive but create lots of enthusiasm among the children. Just like adults, young patients also are responsible for referrals. They say to their friends, "My dentist gave me this!" These children then go to their parents and request the same dentist because of the great prizes. Never underestimate the power of children and the influence they exert on their parents.

All doctors should give away floss, toothbrushes, and other dental aids to their patients. Pinching pennies in these areas is false economy. The hygienist should be able to say, "Mr. Scott, here is your new toothbrush and a sample of floss. Please think of us each day when you use them."

I once believed that having the doctor's name imprinted on toothbrushes and pens bordered on "tacky," until I was out of town and realized I had forgotten to pack my toothbrush. A dental friend presented me with a toothbrush of the type he gives his patients on their first visit (complete with his name and telephone number). Every time I used that toothbrush, the imprinted name reminded me of a pleasant visit to his office. Minor messages work. Giving away imprinted brushes is effective.

Marketing Steps

To formulate a marketing campaign, you need to organize the approach and plan the implementation. Be sure to budget the cost of the program. Many marketing ideas can be expensive with little return, while others will bring in new patients for a small investment.

1. Outline the office marketing objective. To what target group (children, young parents, middle-aged business people, workers, or senior citizens) does the office want to appeal? Each target group responds differently to different messages.
2. Ask for the staff's input on marketing ideas. If it is a team approach, the ideas are more readily implemented.
3. Use the "rifle approach" for the target group the office wants to attract. Select one idea at a time to try. Some offices use the "shotgun" approach, which means they

try every marketing idea they hear about and end up with a mixed message and a confused consumer — the patient.

Following is a list of internal and external marketing ideas I enjoy sharing with doctors and staff. Not all ideas work in every practice. But from the wide variety presented, most practices should find something appropriate.

Marketing Ideas (Children)

1. **Tooth Fairy Membership Kit.** Included is a toothbrush, a tooth chest for lost primary teeth, a tooth fairy bravery badge, and other assorted prizes.
2. **No Cavities Club or Sparkling Smile Club.** Take an instant photo of all child patients who have a cavity-free visit. Place their photo on the "No Cavity Club" bulletin board. As the board fills up, remove the oldest photos and mail them to the patients with a note from the dentist or a staff member.
3. **Prescription for Free Milkshake.** Every time a child patient leaves the office, write a special prescription on a preprinted child-like prescription pad. Arrange ahead of time with your local ice cream store to do this.

> Rx· Dispense one free milkshake (any flavor) to
> _____ for being a great patient today.
> Signed: Dr._____

4. **Calling the Tooth Fairy.** After a child has an extraction, call the parent back to the treatment room. The doctor (chairside) picks up a telephone receiver and personally tells the tooth fairy she should go by the child's house to pick up a tooth tonight. The parents talk about this longer than the surprised child!
5. **Stuffed Animal Drawing.** Each child patient places his or her name in a fishbowl or box for a monthly drawing for a stuffed animal. Take a photo of the child receiving the prize for the office bulletin board or newsletter. The child will boast to friends about the prize that was won from the dentist.

6. **Balloons, Stickers, Rings, and Other Prizes.** Children love prizes and look forward to their visit to the dentist if they get to dig through the toy chest or put a nickel (provided by the office) into the prize machine.
7. **Preschool Tours.** Offer tours of the office to local preschools. Have the children take a ride in the chair, select a prize, and receive a toothbrush during their visit. Make an impression of each child's thumb, and give it to the child before he or she leaves.

Marketing Ideas (General)

1. **New-Patient Welcome Letter.** This should be short and only "welcome to our practice," not a combination welcome and office policy letter. It also is nice to include an appointment card, a map of the office location, and the patient registration form that will need to be completed at the first appointment.
2. **Thank-You Note for Referrals.** Patients who refer patients should be appreciated. "Behavior that is appreciated is repeated." Repeated referrals should be appreciated with a small gift such as a flower in a bud vase with a complimentary note. Other gifts include a lunch for two, show or game tickets, an engraved pen, or a leather accessory.
3. **Flowers.** Any marketing idea can be carried to extremes. Rather than give flowers to every patient every day, I feel flowers should be reserved for special occasions. There is such an occasion in almost every month. On Valentine's Day, for instance, give a long-stemmed red rose and a piece of fern wrapped in green tissue to each patient—even the men. (They can pretend they stopped at the florist on the way home.) Every staff member should also get a rose.

    Call the florists in town to get the best price for a small arrangement delivered to the office every Monday morning. Later in the week, while the flowers are still fresh, choose one patient who has a special need (a family member in the hospital, an anniversary, guests over that evening, or a new baby and give the flowers away.

4. **24-Hour-a-Day Availability.** An answering service or a call forwarding or answering device with remote control lets the doctor be available 24 hours a day. In building a new practice, this availability is essential. In an established practice, it is good public relations.

5. **Local Hotel Dentist.** Many hotels and motels welcome an on-staff dentist for guests who may suffer a dental emergency while at their facility. Leaving the office number with the front desk staff can bring in emergencies (some after hours).

6. **Lecture at PTA and Other Civic Meetings.** Becoming a guest lecturer has proven a good practice-builder for dentists. Develop a half-hour talk on cosmetic dentistry or any interesting topic and leave a professional card for those who may need additional information or a dentist.

7. **Newsletters.** If the office is computerized, a quarterly newsletter mailing list is easy to prepare. For the noncomputerized office, type the master mailing list on adhesive labels. Reproduce the master label list by photocopying the master list each quarter onto blank labels. Each time the business staff types a new ledger card, a new label is typed on the sheet of master labels. A newsletter should be a team effort. Each member of the staff should volunteer for a section such as "Hygiene Tips," "Sugar-Free Recipes," "Insurance Update," "Children's Corner," "On the Road Again" (continuing education courses attended), or "Patient Awareness Tips." The newsletter should be typeset for a professional look. If you have a specialty practice, send the newsletter to general dentists in the area. At dental meetings, ask other practice personnel who publish newsletters to add your office to their complimentary mailing list.

8. **Call Patients at Night.** Call patients in the evening to see how well they are doing after their visit that day. Do not say you are checking for *problems*.

9. **Business Cards for the Staff.** Team members cannot be enthused about "their" office if they do not feel impor-

tant. Staff business cards can be a great marketing tool if used as intended. If each staff member has a personal business card, giving them away becomes a matter of habit.

The staff should take them everywhere they go. For example, when staff go to the cleaners or on any other personal errand and the service person asks "May I have your name and telephone number?", the staff member can pull out a card and leave it. At banks and grocery stores, when the clerks ask for identification, the staff member can give the necessary identification and leave a card as well. Using cards effectively is a habit everyone can develop.

In designing staff business cards, use the same image for the entire office. If the office has a logo, use it on staff cards. The staff member's name and title should be in the center. The address should be preceded by the doctor's name.

10. **Telephone in Reception Room.** A telephone in the reception room for patients' use serves two purposes: (1) it saves the receptionist many interruptions per day when patients ask to use the telephone and (2) it is a nice amenity for patients to use while they are waiting. Some suggestions with a reception room telephone are (1) make sure it is restricted for local outgoing calls only, (2) place a phone book near the phone, and (3) a sticker on the phone should read, "Please limit calls to three minutes or less."

11. **Baby Gifts for New Mothers.** Any time there is a new baby in a family, a prospective new patient has been born. Giving a baby toothbrush, a teething ring, or some other type of baby item is another way of saying "We care."

Marketing Ideas (Specialists)

1. **Treat the General Practitioner and Staff for Reduced Fees.** The general practice staff should feel good enough about the specialist to recommend that person without hesitation.

2. **Help a New General Practitioner Get Started.** The new dental team will always remember the kindness.

3. **Complimentary Photo of Patient in an Ortho Practice.** Early in the treatment, send the patient a certificate for a complimentary portrait. Upon completion of treatment, the patient can have a portrait made of the new smile. The person will talk about it throughout the treatment period.

4. **Give a Present to Patients on Debanding.** The female patients can receive roses, and the male patients might like show tickets.

5. **Sponsor a Little League Team.** Have the team picture in the office. Staff can attend games to cheer the team.

Marketing the practice is definitely a team effort. Marketing from the inside out is most effective because patients perceive the practice by what they see and feel after they arrive. Projecting the best image is a matter of caring how the patient feels.

Dentistry really can be fun, exciting, and rewarding — for patients, dentists, and staff — if everyone in the office becomes personally involved and committed. Managing a dental office is a cinch when a team attitude prevails.

Winning teams are not accidents. They are carefully assembled; they communicate well with each other and their patients, and they appreciate the importance of their various roles. Winning teams strive to perfect their skills and find pleasure in their accomplishments. Winning teams are people-oriented, positive, mindful of production, and enthusiastic.

This book has been about building a winning team. Steps have been outlined, techniques have been described, and examples have been offered. It's improbable that any one dental office would ever adopt all the ideas presented in this book. Even though the ideas have been field-tested and proven valid, each dental office must select the tactics that are best suited for it and for those it serves.

More important, however, are the needs for all the office's personnel — doctors and staff alike — to set goals and work together toward attaining them, to trust and respect one another, and to appreciate and share each with the other. These are the real secrets of teamwork, job happiness, and success.

Index